LAUGHING, N

LAUGHING,
NOT LAUGHING

Edited by

Catherine Merriman

Honno AUTOBIOGRAPHY

Published by Honno
'Ailsa Craig', Heol y Cawl, Dinas Powys
Bro Morgannwg, CF6 4AH

First impression 2004

British Library Cataloguing in Publication Data.

A catalogue record for this book is available from the British Library.

ISBN 1 870206 62 2

Published with the financial support of the Arts Council of Wales

Cover design by Chris Lee
Cover photograph: Gen Nishino/taxi/gettyimages

Typeset and printed in Wales by
Dinefwr Press, Llandybïe.

Contents

Some of the above author names are pseudonyms.

*This anthology also includes work by Sandra Mackness,
Anita Rowe, Barbara Michaels, Jane Blank,
Bethan Gwanas, Justine Curgenven.*

Introduction

I am not an authority on female sexuality. Nor am I an expert on women's social history. I am a fiction writer with an interest in gender issues, originally trained as a sociologist, who has been habitually disdainful of media representations of women's sexual experience, seeing them as either wishful male views, or determined by 'what sells' – that is, concentrating on the romantic, sensational, titillating or problematic – and not by what is truthful. A problem with this view, however, has been that I could never have said with confidence what, exactly, was 'truthful'. Thus, when invited in early 2001 to edit a collection for Honno on a theme of my choice, and aware that collections of women's autobiographical writings have been successful for them in the past, I suggested the non-fiction theme of women's sexual experience. To my delight Honno, after some discussion of practicalities (related to the sensitivity of the subject matter), decided that such a collection would have great interest and value.

Readers will note that the project has taken considerable time from inception to publication – this is simply because it's taken this long to amass enough contributions. (And if we had not offered anonymity I doubt we would have had a volume even now.) Despite media suggestions to the contrary, personal sexual experience is clearly still very much a private matter. Having said that, many of our contributors expressed in their covering letters great enthusiasm for the project – from gratified amazement to urgent encouragement.

The twenty-six pieces we have collected here cannot

pretend to be representative of Welsh women's experience of sex. Indeed, they are most unlikely to be. Women who do not or cannot express themselves on paper will not be here. Nor, I would guess, are women for whom sex is quite unimportant. Women writers are bound to be over-represented. Contributors were offered anonymity (from me, as editor, and any readership, though not from Honno) and the only hard information passed on to me for every piece was the age group of the author. So I have a very partial knowledge of who in fact responded. But 'representativeness' doesn't actually matter, particularly since, mindful of falling into the same 'what sells' trap as others, I have striven to be as inclusive as possible. I make no apology for the fact that some of the pieces are not great literature. Contributors weren't asked for great literature, they were asked for honesty. (All the same, some are beautifully written.) I excluded only those submissions that didn't stick to what was asked for. The brief was a piece written to the theme *My Experience of Sex* which, whilst not expected to be comprehensive, was expected, whatever aspect or area of sexual experience was dealt with, to be factual and honest. Thus I excluded fictional treatments and poetry, hearsay accounts of the experiences of others (every word counted in the brief, including *My*), a few pieces where the sexual experience was not the focus (though it featured) and pieces where the narrator had written an account of a sexual experience, but with so little surrounding context that the result was de-personalized: just a description in a vacuum. I wanted women to be present in their essays and stories, and to hear their voices. What we have ended up with are some pieces that describe in detail a very specific sexual event, others that attempt a broad-brush sexual 'life history', and the rest lying somewhere between these extremes.

If one of our editorial anxieties was that autobiographical pieces focusing on just one aspect of women's lives (rather than a historical period, say) would lack variety, these fears proved groundless. The voices in these pieces, and what they have to say, vary enormously: from the matter-of-fact, even peremptory, to the most intensely self-searching. In their sexual lives women reveal themselves variously as: predatory, worldly-wise, innocent, knowing, lacking in confidence, confident, warm, cool, romantic, unromantic . . . Some contributors have written essays; others have dramatised their accounts. All are interesting. Some are funny, some are sad, some informative, and some, as in those where the writer seems to be achieving self-awareness even as she writes, deeply affecting. I felt privileged to read them all.

By one of those common coincidences, while I was immersed in reading manuscripts the *Observer* newspaper published as a special supplement the results of their own commissioned sex survey *(The Uncovered Poll,* Oct. 2002). This had the subtitle *Everybody's at it: find out how often, who with and if we're doing it right.* Whilst this was not uninteresting (as entertainment, if nothing else) it seemed to me to exemplify precisely how deficient statistics and summary are at illuminating certain subjects. To know that the 'average Briton has sex eight times a month', for instance, is fairly meaningless except perhaps as a marker besides which half the population are expected to feel smug, and the rest deprived or inadequate. It tells us nothing about what that sex is like, nor how it relates to the person experiencing it. (To say nothing of who this 'average couple', in a diverse population, might be, nor how 'having sex' is defined. Penetration? Surely not. Attainment of orgasm? Mutual? Who knows.)

True illumination of a subject such as sexual experience cannot come from the collated results of surveys, or any summarized facts and figures. It would be like asking parents what parenthood is like based on how many children they have, at what ages they had them, which schools the children attended and what exam results were achieved. This would tell us nothing about the really important stuff: what parenthood *feels* like, how it affects a mother or father, and alters their inner as well as their outer lives. Real understanding comes either from personal experience, or from the detailed, honest, personal accounts of others. So it is, surely, with our sexual lives. Thus, while this collection as a whole cannot claim to represent the range of sexual experience of women in Wales, this is immaterial, since we are not seeking to present 'average' or 'typical' results. We are presenting personal accounts. Just one would have value. Twenty six is riches.

And, since we are not looking for summary results, I am reluctant to express here too many conclusions of my own that are drawn from the whole collection. I'll just say that, among many insights gained, I was left with three abiding and connected convictions. First, that even 'minor' inappropriate sexual experiences in childhood can have profound and longstanding impact into our adult lives, but that, secondly, amelioration or change in this impact (recovery, reorientation, revelation leading to self-development) is clearly possible. I thought this latter point a heartening find. The third conclusion is to repeat what I mentioned earlier: that despite the much more open times, reticence on personal sexual matters is still very much the norm, and this clearly leaves many women feeling 'on their own' regarding their sexual lives. This alone-ness, of course, can make them vulnerable. This book is perhaps a small step towards addressing this issue.

So, returning to my original impetus for the book, do I think this collection has provided me with the truth about women's sexual experience? Well, no, because there clearly isn't any one single 'truth'. What it has done is open my eyes to the fact that there are a multitude of individual, varied truths; and I shall certainly be much warier in future about making generalisations on the subject. For this reason I have deliberately made no attempt to sort what follows into subject matter within the overall theme, or indeed shape the collection in any way in terms of content. I have ordered the pieces simply into age group of author, starting with the oldest (60s and over) and continuing through the decades until the youngest (20s). We received no contributions from anyone under twenty. Some of the pieces have been edited for readability and some trimmed, but nothing of substance has been omitted or added, and all edits have been approved by the author. The reader may note that there is not an exact match between the author names as listed on the Contents page and those in the Details on Contributors. This is because of the different levels of anonymity offered to authors. Some were happy to be named on their pieces and in the Notes; others did not wish to be named anywhere in the volume and used pseudonyms or 'Anon'; others were happy to be named as contributors, but not to have their pieces identified as theirs.

I am confident that readers will find this a fascinating and unputdownable book. Thanks for this must go to our contributors, who not only had the courage to pen their pieces to begin with, and trust us with their explorations and confidences, but have endured a long wait to see their efforts in print. I and Honno would like to express our sincere gratitude to them. I'm sure they will agree, after reading the book, that it has been tremendously worth while.

And I would like to add personal thanks to Gwenllïan Dafydd, Janet Thomas and Lindsay Ashford of Honno for their unwavering support. It was Gwenllïan who seconded my original proposal and got the project off the ground, and Janet and Lindsay whose organisational skills and enthusiasm saw the undertaking through. Working with Honno has, as usual, been a real pleasure. My thanks go too to Katie Gramich, who read the manuscript at an early stage, and whose keen eye and positive, constructive comments were very much appreciated.

Catherine Merriman 2003

60s+

*'I hope I shall never become
too old to feel desire.'*

Brazen Hussies

SARAH JONES

Twenty-one and still a virgin. Can you believe that? In the year 1963? Was it all right to do it because the permissive society prevailed? I didn't dare ask my Mum.

He was lovely. His name was Owen. When I was sixteen, I had a crush on him. I watched him speaking at the School Literary Society. The balloon debate rumbled on as I gazed at him with covert admiration. His hair was light brown, curly. He was three years older than me. They said he went out with one of the prefects. I was so gawky. Embarrassed at being tall. Curious about the feelings stirring in me when I looked at Owen. Wondering what it would be like if he were to touch me. One day he cycled past my house when I was just opening the gate, balancing books in my arms. Blushing. I was on my way to the lending library. It was a summer's evening. He saw me and smiled. He cycled on. I walked on, wondering and hoping. When I got to the library he wasn't there. I chose books that I had no intention of reading because my brain was kicking up a storm that was seething inside me.

My knowledge of sex had been obtained in two ways. When I was at primary school there'd been a doctor's daughter in my class. She gave us a fairly accurate explanation of the reproductive process. But what I read in Mum's library books, sneaked from her bedside table whilst she was watching television, was more titillating. Under the smokescreen of Radio Luxembourg I read avidly. I read about a landlady, a widow who wore French knickers and Californian Poppy

3

scent and who took her lodgers into her bed. There was a lot of wriggling and panting and poking. Arching of backs and wet kissing. I was turned on even though I didn't know it was called that.

When I joined the Sixth Form one girl smuggled in a copy of *Lady Chatterley's Lover* and our lunch-breaks were spent reading 'those passages'. We were trying to understand Advanced Level Sex without the benefit of coursework. We giggled about forget-me-nots and pubic hair. We discussed what it must be like to do it. Imagined mouths kissing, tongues seeking, fingers probing, knees bumping. How terrible it would be to become an unmarried mother.

Owen had left school, presumably gone on to University. I completed A Levels, did brilliantly in one but bombed otherwise. I completed a college course and took a job at Cardiff Airport. I wore a blue uniform. I was no longer gawky. One night, I was just coming off shift when Owen turned up. He stood in front of the counter and told me he'd noticed me when he'd been collecting some friends who'd been on a package holiday to Majorca. He wondered if I'd like to go out with him for a coffee. I liked.

It was so delicious, what he did to me later in the car. Of course I let him. I'd known him for years, hadn't I? We would just feel each other. But his finger was rhythmic and insistent and I was moist and warm and welcoming, wriggling out of my pants. My breasts took on a life of their own. They were pushing themselves at him. Brazen hussies. When I came, I shuddered and sighed and shivered but Owen quickly placed my hand on his hard cock and showed me what I should do. He was silky and smooth and big and I wanted to feel him inside me but I knew we mustn't do it. Then he removed my hand and rolled on top of me, rubbing his cock against me. And I opened my legs wide for him.

Should he have asked permission? Would it have made any difference? He pushed against the girl and entered the woman and I turned my head and felt the sharp pain slice through me whilst he nuzzled soft lips against my neck. Then he was thrusting in and out. And this time I knew there was something more valuable for the having. The fingering had been lovely but this was the jewel in the crown.

I let the sensation lap over me and dissolve my bones and my heart and my brain as I writhed against him and sucked on his tongue and wound my fingers through the curly hair at the nape of his neck. We moved and rocked together. Masters of the art at the first attempt. Go on. Go on. Lovely, lovely fuck. You mustn't stop now. You can't stop now. Fuck me hard. Do it. Do it. But he groaned and pulled out. Spasm after spasm. He came over the car seat. I wound my fingers around his wetness but instinctively just cradled him in my hand. He kissed my mouth then bent and inserted his tongue just between my legs, flicking and licking amongst the intricacies. I was surprised but still hovering on the brink. I completed the roller-coaster ride to my orgasm, real and wonderful, as it swelled and exploded and made me cry out in the steamy cocoon of the car.

Owen laughed. Owen cuddled me. Owen said he'd unlocked my treasures and that he would hold the key to them for ever more. He said he loved me and no other man would go where he had been. Six weeks later he dumped me. Moved on. I was forgotten. But the legacy he left me would be with me forever. Still is. I hope I shall never become too old to feel desire.

Passion Killers

ANNE COLLEDGE

Sex, we dare not say the word when we were children growing up in Ruabon, a small village in North Wales, where I was born in 1939. We children spelt out s-e-x, and said, don't mention it, just say the initial, then we won't get into trouble. Even 'knickers' counted as a dirty word to our mothers.

I don't remember any sex education at the Grammar school I went to. The girls' school occupied Nissan huts, reputed to be from the First World War. The boys' school was a brick building next door and we girls spent every spare moment parading across their playground, which linked the two schools, pretending to be oblivious to the boy's stares. The only time the two sexes met officially was at the Sixth Form Christmas party held in the boys' gym, which was so cold that the masters' wives attended in winter coats. We were given ballroom dancing lessons in November ready for the party. We learnt the Quick Step and spent hours practicing, shouting one, two, three, together and arguing which girl went backwards, taking the man's part.

Our school uniform was a bottle green gymslip with large pleats, tied, like a sack in the middle, with a belt. Erotic it was not and in no way invited passionate interest. The more forward girls hitched their skirts up but this was soon forbidden. Part of the uniform was our *directoire* knickers, bottle green, of course, which were voluminous and could be pulled up under our arms and stretched down to our knees. Our vests were home-knitted in scratchy Welsh wool, two plain two purl, and with the liberty bodices it was hard to find our bodies never mind worry about them.

My friend, Ann, and I did graduate to boyfriends at about eleven and the four of us went to the Presbyterian Chapel Band of Hope on Mondays. We used to leave notes under stones saying 'We love you' but no one knew who loved whom. At the Christmas party at the Chapel we played Spin the Knife and had to kiss the nearest boy. We also went into the porch for dare kisses.

At eighteen I left the village to go to college at Cambridge. My Welsh accent was so strong that people could not understand what I said. I wrote home to my mother about the Coffee Bars, popular then, and told her someone had asked me out for dinner. I got a letter by return of post saying, 'Do not go out to dinner with men. If they pay for your dinner they will only want One Thing.' I did not know what to write home about after that in case it sent her into a flap of worry.

At that time there were eight men to every woman at Cambridge, which I loved. In the beginning I went out with lots of different men. I think it was the effect of being so repressed at home.

My fellow students and I spent the whole of our spare time discussing 'How Far to Go' with our boyfriends. We drew up maps of our bodies with lines beyond which no one must trespass. Pregnancy was the main worry and wanting a meaningful relationship. 'I was brought up Welsh Non-Conformist,' I would explain to the men I went out with as I legged it safely home.

Rumours went round the college that a student had been sent to Sweden by her rich father for an abortion. This was a great scandal.

I was invited to the May Ball, which went on all night and ended with breakfast at Grantchester, and had to get permission from my parents. The letter came back with an unequivocal, 'No, you can't go. No decent woman stays out all night.' Desperate to go and trying to make it seem respectable, I wrote back that the Bishop would be attending. They replied that Bishops were worse than anyone. But they did relent and grudgingly gave permission for me to go. The rugby club song went, 'Three hundred virgins went to the Ball, None came back at all.' Anyway my partner and I decided we had better not have sexual intercourse, so at least one virgin returned.

Years later my mam, who was born in 1902 and was then ninety-two, said out of the blue, 'I wish we'd let you go to that dance in Cambridge.'

'I did go, and times were different then,' I said.

Mam told me she worried about getting pregnant all her married life, all spent in Ruabon. I was a mistake, and they could not afford more children. She married at twenty-eight years old because they had to save enough money to furnish their house before they married, since women did not work outside the home afterwards.

I was twenty-two when I married. In those days it was the only way you could have a sex life. I went to the Family Planning in Chester to be fitted with a Dutch Cap. 'This one has holes in it,' the doctor announced, giving me a warning look. I was to practice using it until the wedding and just before the date, which I was grilled about, I suppose to stop any unmarried sex, I would be given one without holes in it.

I was married for fourteen years and then divorced. Looking back I do not think the strict restrictions on sex before marriage did us any harm. It gave us time and space to grow up without too many worries, although maybe it caused us to marry young.

After my divorce I decided to tag on to the tail end of the permissive society, but that is another story and needs to be anonymous. Who says you can't teach an old dog new tricks? Although I think you never throw off your early training. The Jesuits said, 'Give me a child under seven years old and I will have them for life.' Anyway, why throw off a good beginning? The morals we were taught at that time were meant to protect us and nothing gives you a better start in life than a good home and loving parents. We also had a strong community in the village and that was good, it gave us roots.

Laughing, Not Laughing

ELIZABETH BAINES

Ray Doyle's van scooped to a halt ahead of me as I walked towards the sunset up the North Road, T S Eliot under my arm.

Ray Doyle was short, boxy, not particularly pretty, a dynamo of energy and anarchy. He drove his van as if it were a plane and the road the air. When he wasn't in his van he walked tipped forward as if in his head he'd already got where he was going, his Dylan-Thomas lock of hair going first. His blue eyes, in their rather puffy sockets, were always laughing silently at some big cosmic joke no one else had yet got.

It was the sixties. I was seventeen, and he was twenty-seven.

He didn't act his age. He and his four adult brothers still lived on the council estate with their parents and cheerfully sent them wild by driving too fast and coming home late and drunk and standing in a row and peeing up the side of the house. I had a problem imagining him working in a tie and collar, which allegedly he did, at the paper mill. In the baths, he and his mate Digger dive-bombed me and my sister Jenny or sneaked up underwater to give us a fright. They would hang about outside afterwards, hair slicked, towels rolled, and invite us for a ride in the van. Or they'd wait for us outside the Crown when they came out of the bar and we came down from the folk club upstairs with all the studenty school-kid types.

Ray Doyle said he was mad on me, and physically he was, but he didn't mind, in fact he thought it a great joke, that I had a *steady boyfriend*, Derek, away at university, who must never find out what was going on.

The road ahead glittered, liquid with sun.

Ray Doyle stuck his head out. He gave a comic's nod at the book beneath my arm. 'Wanna hop in?'

I shook my head. 'I've got an exam tomorrow.'

A-level Poetry. My passport out of this small northern English town and life with my free-fisted Dad.

Ray Doyle chuckled, showing his gappy little teeth.

I hopped in.

Derek was my soulmate.

I'd met him in chapel when I was fifteen years old. I looked up towards the gallery and there he was with his square-cut jaw, in his narrow trousers, a nifty tweed jacket and the Rupert-Bear type waistcoat that was just then in fashion, and intellectual horn-rimmed specs (*The Professor*, Ray Doyle called him though he'd never even met him, always with a chuckle). Derek's specs flashed; he looked out across the domed chapel. I saw from his gaze that his mind, like mine, was bent on better places and higher things, and I fell slap-bang in love.

He had a father who was a verbal bully, just as mine was a physical one. He told me he'd sucked his thumb till he was twelve years old and I cried, 'So did I!' and the shame we'd each suffered over this floated clean away through the blossom above us, where we lay on the grass with our bikes thrown down.

He didn't touch me when he didn't have to.

I felt so *loved* by this. After all the beatings from my father, I felt so *cherished*, so *respected* by a boy, a man, who seemed so in awe of my personal limits and the integrity of my body. He was too aware of the importance of touching, I thought, to squander such a thing.

Of course, he held my hand in the chapel youth club, since this was the accepted mode of conduct for a couple *going out together*, a signal to potentially interested other parties to *lay off*. And of course, by the same token, we snogged publicly, along with everyone else, on the bus coming home from the evangelical rallies, but these were mere rituals imposed from outside: as the others tumbled, flushed, onto the bus and onto each other to relieve the excess erotic force with which God had just moved them to transfigure a couple of hundred souls, I would turn to Derek with a sense of affection and duty rather than lust, and a residual resentment at the ritual nature of the action and the social imperative (for if couples were seen on the bus not snogging then they'd be presumed to have *finished* and others would *move in*).

The truly erotic time for me with Derek was when the bus had dropped us off in town and he walked me home up the North Road. *Then* he didn't hold my hand. He'd walk beside me intently questioning the existence of the god we were meant to have just been on a mission to convince others of, looking up at the expanding universe to support his case, and imparting to me his developing socialist philosophy. This was when I felt romanced. This was how I felt he really touched me: with his mind.

And then he went to university, and I pined. I loved Derek most of all when he wasn't even there.

'How's the Professor?' said Ray Doyle with a chuckle, as I hopped in for one last time, laughing of course but protective of Derek and refusing to answer. I slid into the seat beside him and into the lithe and desirable body I always had in this van (checking that my book was stowed safe by my side).

For one last time we screamed up the North Road, past the estate where Dad would be tinkering in the garage unaware I was doing the very thing the possibility of which he'd always meant to beat out of me, tearing out between the fields where hares with giant elongated shadows sat stock-still, the sun like red neon in their ears. One last time we swung into the woods and stopped in the clearing, one last time Ray Doyle pulled the handbrake and turned and looked me over with a silent awed 'Phew.'

This time he said, 'That Derek. That Professor. He's no idea about you.'

Well, that was true.

When Derek told me he'd sucked his thumb he added with a meaningful grin, 'Of course, I stopped at the age of twelve because I discovered other, better pleasures.'

I stared.

He laughed, kindly and amused.

He thought me an innocent.

I didn't like to say, I never told him, that I was amazed he hadn't masturbated before the age of twelve.

When I'm five years old, while my mother is packing for our move from South Wales to Rhyl, the neighbour's eight-year-old daughter brings me to orgasm beneath a blanket on the lawn.

Such a sweet and unexpected pleasure.

And forbidden: she tells me that. Whoever taught *her* has told her that.

She leans over me, her face close to mine, hot beneath the blanket, belligerent and urgent, her whisper strangely coarse. 'You must never, ever tell! Not your Mummy, no one!'

How can this be? That such a sweet and melting pleasure, such a thrill in my deep inner core, is a matter for shame? A matter for secrecy. It cuts me off from my mother: for the first time ever, the bond between us is tainted by secrecy and shame.

It makes me so lonely.

But it's such a sweet slipping pleasure. The sensation such consolation for the shame. And such consolation for the sudden changes in our life: the gloomy flat with its tobacco-brown paint on the walls, the smears of neon on the concrete in the strange town through the window, our mother's sighs and sad withdrawal over her heavily-pregnant frame, our father's darkening moods and the fact that now when we're naughty he beats us.

'Line up,' he will say to us, when we've been bad. *Line up*, as if we're a regiment or a gang, but there's only the two of us, me and Jenny, six and four years old.

He has placed the wooden chair in the centre of the lino, athletic and one-handed, setting it down gracefully with hardly a sound. A line of light shines on the lino through the legs of the chair. He sits himself down on it, ceremonious, his huge stocky legs obliterating the line of light.

We are half-undressed for bed. My bare skin cringes. We have been dreading this for hours. It is hours since our mother promised to tell our father we've been naughty, and we have exhausted ourselves with anxiety, looking out through the window for his black Austin to appear in the street below. We have been motionless with dread since at last the door boomed shut in the cave of the building below and his heavy footsteps rose towards us.

There's a frightened scuffle now, as we beg each other to go first. I know I shouldn't be begging Jenny, she's littler than me, but if I go first I'll get the brunt of his anger, whereas because she's littler she won't, he'll hold off, and then when he gets to me he'll have lost some steam.

He shuts us up. He decides, as always. Me, the eldest, the ringleader.

I can't make myself go. I know I must, but I can't, my legs are moving backwards of their own accord.

He booms evenly, 'Every bloody backward step you take, you'll get an extra bloody smack.'

And then there's the sensation of diving underwater as I'm propelled across his knee, lungs congested, blood running to my head, and the stinging blows descend.

And after this, the sight of his huge hand coming down on Jenny's plump little four-year-old bum.

And then the swollen waterlogged feeling as we lie in our

shared bed, the songs sobbing from the dance halls and amusement arcades outside, my arm around Jenny for comfort, the salty taste of my own badness on my tongue, the shape of my badness on the sheets.

I teach my consoling secret to Jenny. When a cousin comes to stay, we teach it to her.

I insist she mustn't tell. I can't guess that though she has a guilty conscience she has none of the caution and fear of consequences our father has already beaten into us. She tells her mother, our aunt.

Her mother tells ours.

In the gloom of our flat, my mother's face seems to me white with shock.

She has challenged us. She has put it obliquely, in a way which, if we are innocent as she has supposed, we'd never have understood.

I understood only too well. I have broken down, the truth bursting out of me through a dam of such tension that I'm flooded not only by horror and shame but also relief.

But there is to be no relief.

It's an early evening in late spring, and I'm sitting in a shaft of sun which blinds me, cuts me off from my mother in the darkness of the flat. I can only see her by moving my head, her face white and disembodied in the gloom. She is slumped in the chair, shattered by childbirth and home-sickness, and by our father's dramatically worsening temper. It seems to me in my guilt that she is silent and slumped with shock.

And I am in shock. That the deepest pleasure of my body could be responsible for causing my Mummy such hurt.

Daddy's right. I am wicked. It is me who poisoned Jenny and our cousin. The really bad one, the really corrupt one, is me.

I say in sudden terror, 'Don't tell Daddy, will you?'

And my mother says no, she won't.

This is so bad she can't tell him. This is so bad there is no knowing what he'd do to us if he found out.

The sun slices through the window and onto the table, cutting through the room like a sword. I look out through the shaft of sun, follow the line of light over the fire-escape rail, across the slate roofs opposite and on over this jangly seaside town where we don't belong, where we're lost.

I promise never to do it again, and I mean it with a fierce passion: I want to rid myself of this poison and corruption.

But I can't stop it. I'm addicted: I need it more. And each time I do it (secretly from Jenny, because I mustn't implicate her now) the guilt and loneliness are sharper and the sense of corruption more deeply seeping. Afterwards, always, I pray to God to forgive me, but then imagine the Lord Jesus at the foot of the bed, his bearded face a mask of censure and sorrow, and my mind freezes up with the sense that I am damned.

I'm corrupt, and I'm sensitised now to the corruption around me. It's everywhere: it sobs and echoes from the dance halls and amusement arcades, it's all along the prom, men with their hands surreptitiously all over girls, couples glimpsed down alleyways, slipped away from the neon dimensions into each other's arms. It's a constant aching slide of men and women together. It's supposed to be secret but it's even advertised on the cinema hoardings, and it always causes grief.

There's the couple my parents know who take me and Jenny for a walk on the prom. It's a windy day and Susan's full skirt kites and Oliver laughs in a way that alerts my corruption-sensitive antennae and I stare. I see that the skin of Oliver's face around his slick black moustache is strangely stiff and opaque, and I realise that he's quite old, older than my parents, let alone Susan.

From a stall on the prom they buy us each a fresh peach, and as we eat them, absorbed, they move away. I look up. Oliver and Susan are locked in a deep embrace.

They are clamped together. With my peach clamped in my mouth, I stare. Susan's body is bent submissively backwards, at odds with the greedy force with which her arm is flung around his neck. He bends above her, domineering, but this contrasts disturbingly with the way the wind troubles his black hair. She squirms subtly, and his mouth moves with little greedy but somehow desperate twitches over hers.

I know in that instant that what they are doing is forbidden.

And then there is the day that Oliver's wife, a skinny sad woman, comes to the flat with her two troubled little boys, en route to Scotland where she's taking them for good.

Affair. I hear my parents whisper the word.

I read it in the paper. There's a picture of a woman in a deep-cut dress which shows off her white shoulders. She has a name from the Bible, *Ruth*, but her nails are long and painted, and she's holding a wine glass, her little finger sticking out the way Susan's does.

The newspaper makes a big point of the fact that she's blonde.

Ellis. Such an ordinary second name, yet there's nothing ordinary about what she's done: taken a gun and murdered the man with whom she has had an *affair.*

She has been sentenced to death.

Bad women, bad girls, who give in to their own corruption, destroy themselves and others. Bad women, bad girls, can get hanged.

Across the alley behind the flat is the back of a pub. Here Jenny and I sit on the yard step and play with scattered bottle tops, putting them into piles of red, yellow, blue and brown. From the impenetrable beer-smelling cave, through the tinkle of glasses, comes a woman's low laugh, lapped immediately by the deeper laughter of men.

The laugh of a woman who goes into pubs, the kind of woman who was hanged.

There's a soft scuffle, and two men come out of the back door, two soldiers in uniforms like prickly blankets with their caps twisted under their epaulettes.

'Hello, Blondie,' says one of them, and he ruffles my hair as if sealing my fate.

From back in the pub comes the woman's laugh again. It swims in the shadows like a lazy fish which could slip away quickly into the depths, or could be caught.

This corrupt thing I do is not my only consolation.

I'm in love all the time – with one boy or man or another: the boy who brings the groceries, the young man who works in the offices downstairs. I have only to be alone for one minute, guarding the pram outside a shop, say, and I'm off into a world of daydream in which my chosen loved one of the moment rescues me from a house on fire or thunders up on a horse like John in *Lorna Doone* to whisk me out of harm's way. This world of daydream is a pure one, of love that's heroic, of altruistic romance. An antidote to my other shameful addiction.

And then I cross a frightening line. One night, for the first time ever, when my corrupt and consoling hand is between my corrupt and craven legs, a daydream enters my head. It flowers beneath my shut eyes, technicolour, lurid, and I'm shocked even as I'm riveted: there's my young male teacher, the person with whom I am currently in love, in a room lit by candles, face down but naked on a couch as I approach to put my hand on his buttocks . . .

Now there can be no doubt I am truly wicked. Seven years old, I lie, drenched in sweet and cloying orgasmic release, but already shrivelling and asking myself where such a shocking vision could have come from. Knowing the answer: from my own corrupt and poisonous brain.

Next day in school I cannot face my teacher. In class, he asks me a question. I stand up to answer. My tongue solidifies, the words stick like a frozen lump in my throat, and in my mind which is supposed to be clever, but which is poisoned and corrupt, the vision reappears. My limbs feel numb. The silence goes on, and my teacher, whose pet I am usually, rolls his eyes and says wearily, 'Sit down!'

He purses his lips with irritation, and for the first time ever – no wonder, after what I have done to him in my head – I am someone who displeases him.

I can't get rid of the vision. I'm addicted to it. That night I replay it as I bring myself to orgasm. But as I lie, replete, afterwards, I am clear: my love for my teacher is tainted, destroyed.

From now on, I know, I must keep the two things separate: this irresistible swooning release of my body and being in love with another.

Ray Doyle thought it the biggest joke of all that I could be so serious about Derek, and never, after all this time, have had sex with him.

Not that I'd had actual sex with Ray Doyle, that wasn't what was going on. Snogging, yes, heavy petting, his hand in my pants (where Derek's had never been), the harsh wool of his trousers with their swollen ridge of penis pushed between my legs.

Well, I couldn't get pregnant, and I didn't trust Durex, there was too much at stake: I had to get out and away from my bullying dad.

And I was keeping myself for Derek, of course.

Ray Doyle laughed, pulled away ruefully as usual when I stopped him going further, chuckled softly into my neck. This was always the moment when I could have relented, pulled him back again, because I felt so *loved*, so *respected* by his male physical reticence – his above anyone's, a guy renowned as a Lothario and whose van on the grass behind us was widely known as the Shaggin' Wagon.

But of course I didn't pull him back again, not tonight

especially, the night before my last exam, the prelude to my escape into the world.

Ray Doyle leaned back over me suddenly, pinned my arms to the grass.

His face was serious. This was different: it was laughing, as much as snogging, that was usually going on with Ray Doyle.

He said seriously, 'Don't do it.'

I tried to struggle up. 'Oh yeah, stick around in this dump of a town!'

He held me pinned. He said softly and urgently, 'I don't mean not go to university. I mean don't stick with that guy Derek.'

I struggled up and he let me.

I thought he was jealous – which was rich, coming from him, the town Casanova. I laughed.

There was nothing possessive in the next thing he said. 'You could have anybody. Go to university. You can have any life you choose. Don't saddle yourself with him.'

I was cross, but I was touched by his mistaken blessing as well, and I sank back, melting, as he slipped his hand between my thighs. It wasn't *snogging* after all, it never was with Ray Doyle, it was slipping into another, warmer dimension, a coming back to myself.

I saw him years later, in the chemist's, on one of my visits back, after I was married to Derek. He was there with a child, a little pale-haired girl of about four, who kept darting around the shop and then slamming into his wiry, knee-crooked legs. His plain face was smashed, pleated with a lurid scar, from one ride round town which had made the local papers by ending where people like my dad had always promised.

He didn't speak to me. He saw me, of course, his whole compact body was sprung with recognition. I thought: he's too embarrassed, by my proving him wrong, back here and married to Derek and happy, after all the one not damaged.

I wanted to speak to him. I wanted to know, about the accident, his marriage, the kid. I wanted to challenge his silence.

But I couldn't.

I couldn't squash a different idea. That what silenced him was horror, that it was horror on his face when I looked back after slipping from his van that last night, safely down the road so that neither Dad nor Derek would find out what had been going on. That he knew then that all through the rest of the swinging sixties and into the so-called liberated seventies I would fail to reconcile my sensuality with being in love. That it would be years before making love with Derek would bring me the sensation I'd only ever had from myself and Ray Doyle.

Neil Beckett was large, boxy, not particularly pretty, a writer with an air of anarchy and a wry sense of humour.

He thought it was a great joke that I was married to a doctor and lived in a suburban house with just less than two point five kids – which was a pretty rude thing to say to someone you've only just met.

I laughed.

I looked away to take my ticket from my wallet. Any second now I'd ditch him, get through the barrier and onto the train and back to my life with Derek, my soulmate, with whom I was living happily ever after, the man I'd waited for years to be with, the man that I loved.

I looked up. I saw nothing. Something enclosed me, a darkness, a warmth, a different dimension. It was moments before I knew it was his kiss and embrace, but already, in my disorientation, I knew I was coming back to myself . . .

Playing the Field

MELANIE GLYN

Casual sex can be very exciting. I didn't discover this until I was forty, so strong was the grip of the old North Wales chapel of my childhood. And at first I wouldn't admit to myself that an affair was purely for sex; I had to pretend to myself I was in love. A lot of women are like that.

I remember being in a crowded nightclub, dancing with a man I'd just met. He was around my age, perhaps a little older, balding and growing a bit of a paunch, but interesting to talk to and with a smile that turned me on. We did old fashioned cheek to cheek stuff while the young things jigged around us. His hand was on my back, warm on the bare skin revealed by my low-backed dress. He was holding me close to him, so close that I could feel his body all the way down, could feel his hardness. It aroused the same thrill in me that I'd felt way back in my teens. My body responded in spite of myself. I pushed against him lightly.

During a brief lull in the cacophony he whispered in my ear, referring to a conversation half an hour before, 'So, you want to go home early?'

'Yes.' I tried to sound as convinced as I had been. The women I had come with were staying out late. But I wasn't just a pleasure seeker like them, was I?

'To sleep? Alone?' His voice was a caress.

'Mm, well, yes.'

He held me at arm's length and stared into my eyes, laughing, sure of himself now. 'But why?'

Two or three drinks earlier I'd felt sure I knew the answer. But now? Why indeed? I was single once more. It was a Friday and I wasn't working next day.

'I've forgotten why.' Now I was laughing too.

'Let's go, then.'

We sought out the others to say goodbye. Jade, who had fancied him first, who was younger, slimmer and prettier than me, fixing us with her bold, blue stare, struck a pose that emphasised the height of her mini skirt and the depth of her décolletage. She grinned, winked and shouted above the music in her broad Valleys accent, 'Going off to fuck, are you then?'

'Keith is seeing me home.' I tried to imagine my chapel hat on and failed. We gave little embarrassed titters and fled.

Walking hand in hand through the cool air of the summer night, I pointed out some of the famous old buildings as we passed. I lived in the city centre, knew it like the back of my hand by now. He was a stranger, here on business for a few weeks. He'd said earlier he was married but separated; there were 'problems'. We strolled through the well-lit main streets in holiday mood.

But as we left the bright lights for the maze of mean streets where I lived the darkness had a different feel. We stepped on in silence broken only by the tapping of my flimsy shoes on the pavement. I knew nothing about this man. He could be a serial killer, the nightmare scenario of every woman with a casual pick-up. Maybe he had his fears too. I could be leading him into a trap where he would be attacked and robbed. My heart beat faster and in a strange way my fear heightened my lust.

Seemed like he felt the same way. He stopped in the dark street and took me in his arms. I slipped mine round his neck and we kissed for the first time, deeply and hotly. As our tongues explored each other's, his hands caressed my body all over. It seemed like an age since anyone had done that and it was so, so sweet. My hands slid down to his bum and pulled his crotch hard against mine. He began to knead one of my breasts softly. Then our hands were everywhere. We stood there feeling each other up like two teenagers with no home to go to. I began to long to take off my dress and feel his naked body against mine.

'Let's get home.' My voice sounded husky and strange. Reluctantly we separated and carried on through the dark streets. It wasn't far, but it seemed so long that we had to stop and kiss and explore each other's bodies again on the way. At last we arrived at my three-storey terrace house and crept upstairs, although there was no one to hear.

'Does anyone else rent any of these rooms?' He looked around.

I shook my head. 'This is my house. My children are grown up and I live alone.' My fears must have totally evaporated.

In the bedroom we flung off our clothes and fell on the bed, our naked limbs entwined. But after all the build-up it was over too quickly. He pulled out just before ejaculating and I didn't come.

'I wish it had gone on longer,' I said, still wanting him. That's one good thing about casual sex; you can just say what you feel without worrying about hurting your partner's feelings.

'I'm sorry, I usually like to take my time too, but I just wanted you too much. Never mind, it'll be better in the morning. I promise.'

I thought I'd never be able to sleep, being too excited, but gradually the warmth of his body against mine, the feeling of his strong arms around me, a feeling I'd missed for so long, lulled me into a sweet, sensual reverie and thence to oblivion.

In the morning we made love again with me on top, riding the wild horse of my desire into the crest of a wave, but as I was about to come he pushed me off just before he came.

'I don't want you to get pregnant.'

'I won't, I have a coil.' I hadn't bothered to have it removed after my marriage ended.

He took a lot of reassuring that it was safe. Only 98% safe? What if I was one of the other 2%? He was obviously a person who liked to be in control. That was probably why he hadn't fancied Jade. She was coming on too strong and he'd wanted someone reluctant he could choose to seduce.

Keith lasted three weeks. After that, I found that he'd somewhat misled me about his relationship with his wife so I stopped seeing him. I couldn't bear the thought of hurting another woman as I'd been hurt in the past. During that time we made love often, and while it was always enjoyable and exciting, I never experienced an orgasm while I was with him. It was always later, when I was alone, reliving our lovemaking in my imagination. There were times when I could come quite spontaneously, without even masturbating, aroused only by mental pictures, scene-playing in my head. I was unable to concentrate on much else during those three weeks, so in a way I was relieved when it was over.

It was in the same nightclub with the same gang, a few months later, that I met Dafydd. He was much younger than me, short, slim, very dark and handsome. In fact, he looked younger than my sons. This time it was not Jade but Mair who had taken a fancy to him. In the ladies' room she told me she'd slept with him at a wild party the previous evening and was looking forward to repeating the experience that night. Young, pretty, but very fat, Mair picked up boyfriends as casually and frequently as hamburgers and cream cakes, yet managed to convince herself that each was the one and only love of her life. Now Dafydd was the heart-throb of the moment, so although I felt very attracted to him and he seemed to feel the same way about me, I decided he was off limits. Too young for me, anyway.

But he had other ideas. This time we were all jiving, so it wasn't a partners thing. Not in a circle dancing round our handbags, either, it was more fluid than that. While Mair kept wriggling and gyrating with remarkable agility for her size, as close as she could get to Dafydd, and I was deliberately doing my own thing some distance away, his steps were taking him little by little away from her and towards me. Eventually he was dancing right in front of me, and taking my hand he whirled me round. Seeing Mair glaring at us, I fanned my face with my hand and mimed going for a drink. He followed me. At the bar I turned on him sternly, trying to make myself heard above the music.

'I wish you'd stay away from me. This is really embarrassing! Mair is going to be very upset. You should be dancing be with her.'

'Why should I be dancing with Mair? She isn't my girlfriend or anything.'

'She seems to think she is.'

He laughed. 'Mair is a great girl. Very clever, witty, good company. But I've never been sexually attracted to fat girls. I fancied her sidekick, that Jade, but she went off with someone else.'

'Didn't you sleep with Mair last night?'

'As a matter of fact, I did. Quite literally. We both happened to be at this party and by 3 a.m. I was shattered. Several folk had crashed out on the floor. Mair and I stretched out on a settee and had a cuddle, which is as far as I go in a room full of people. Five minutes later I was dead to the world. At 7.30 I woke to the sound of her snores, slipped off my two inches of space, drove home and had a shower.'

Sounded as if Mair had been weaving her usual fantasies. But I didn't want to cause trouble so I said I was tired and going home. He offered to see me to my car, I said no thanks, but he came along anyway and I didn't want to create a scene. Mair and Jade glared as we went out together.

So when we reached the car and he said he had no intention of going back to the club as he needed to find a bed for the night, I thought I might as well be hanged for a sheep! He was very attractive, after all. His eyes were so dark they looked opaque, like two pieces of coal, no difference between iris and pupil.

But I was annoyed about him following me out to the car. I still thought of Keith as having been a brief love affair rather than a casual pick up and didn't want to think of myself as being promiscuous. I felt different from Jade and Mair even though I sometimes went around with them. Hadn't intended picking a quarrel with them, though. They were friends of a sort. My feelings were very ambivalent and I must have been giving out mixed messages. I told Dafydd he could have my spare room for the night. When we got to my house I felt glad I'd told him that because I'd gone off the idea of maybe sleeping with him. Something had changed in the atmosphere between us. Sensing some hidden hostility in him, my feeling of attraction had evaporated. He didn't seem inclined to chat, said he was tired, so I showed him the bathroom and the spare room. I went in to close the curtains and as I turned to go out again he barred my way and put his hands on my shoulders. It was the first time he'd touched me. I stood still, waiting to see if that sexual magic would recur. Part of me wanted him to do something that would turn me on. He bent his head and gave me a brief, perfunctory peck on the lips. Then he opened the top button of my blouse. I froze.

Pushing him aside, I strode out and said 'Goodnight' with determined finality. I caught a brief glimpse of his black eyes flashing angrily as I closed the door. Soon I was in my own bed in the room just across the landing, listening out for any sound, feeling anxious and fearful. What a fool I'd been to take a complete stranger into my house yet again. It must have seemed as if I'd been leading him on and now I'd left him feeling angry and frustrated. What if he came into my room in the night? I'd rather die than go through with any sexual activity I didn't feel like. Stupid, perhaps, but it's a matter of integrity, of self-respect. My ex husband had used me, but no way would I let a passing stranger have his way with me just because he felt like it. It had to be mutual. Why that cold little peck instead of a proper kiss, I wondered? AIDS had just been discovered: was he afraid it could be caught through French kissing? Or maybe he was one of those men who need women for sex but don't really like us. Dafydd wasn't a big man, but he'd looked grim as he barred my way in the bedroom. A sort of power ploy. I didn't go for that at all. I'd let my ex mistreat me in so many ways. I'd walked out vowing never to let a man bully me again. Deciding to stay awake all night, just in case, I promptly fell asleep.

The first rays of the sun found me in a relaxed, cheerful mood. I immediately thought of my guest across the landing. Remembering how good-looking he was, how charming he'd seemed in the night club, I began to feel randy and lay there debating whether I should look in on him. Our chaste night seemed so ridiculous now.

Then I heard his door open, footsteps going downstairs. The front door slammed. Damn! I cursed myself for being a fool. He'd only wanted one thing and hadn't got it, so he'd gone. And it was only 7.30. Well, what had I wanted with a man young enough to be my son? And I hadn't got it either.

Five minutes later I thought, no point lying around regretting it now, might as well get up and have a shower. I took off my nightie and slipped into my dressing gown. As I was crossing the landing towards the bathroom Dafydd's voice came from behind the closed door of the spare bedroom.

'Melanie?'

Surprised, I opened the door. He was sitting up in bed, smiling, looking good enough to eat for breakfast with his sparkling white teeth, his brown torso emerging from the bedclothes. He'd somehow managed to wash, clean his teeth and comb his hair without my hearing a thing. And he must have crept silently back upstairs after slamming the front door. He patted the bed beside him. 'Come here and talk to me.'

I sat down, laughing. 'Did you sleep well?'

'You're kidding! I didn't sleep a wink. Did you?'

'Yes, I slept just fine – until I heard the front door slam.'

'And how did you feel then?'

'Disappointed, and a bit randy,' I admitted.

He pulled the bedclothes back to reveal the rest of his smooth, brown body and an enormous erection. I began to open the silk robe I was wearing, but he put out his hand. 'No, leave it on and come in here as you are.'

Why do men always prefer partly clothed to naked? Just as well, really, for a forty year old who's had four children. The state of my body by no means matched his, and I was grateful not to have to reveal my stretch marks straight off. I felt flattered that he'd gone to so much trouble to seduce a woman of forty.

'Kiss me properly this time.'

He did so with great expertise.

We spent an enjoyable hour and he let me go on top, but I didn't come. Of course I didn't have to pretend to have an orgasm – that's another good thing about casual sex. With my husband in the last few years of our marriage I'd had to pretend all the time. After a while this made me feel that it couldn't really happen any more and it didn't. It made me go off him in a big way and then he found someone else. If he hadn't, and if we'd had help, maybe we could have worked things out. Who knows?

Why did I have to pretend? I've thought a lot about this. When we first married I was seventeen and pregnant. We'd been going out with each other since we were at school and he was my first boyfriend. At first the sex was great, but for years I had to pretend I didn't really enjoy it, that I only did it to please him! He apparently thought that nice girls shouldn't like sex. And that was in the fifties, believe it or not. A lot of men thought that in those days. But throughout the sixties and seventies fashions in sexual morality changed, and my husband suddenly wanted me to behave like a nympho-maniac. Whereas at one time I used to have grit my teeth and not let a sound escape when I had an orgasm, now I was not only allowed to make a noise, but he actually got annoyed if I didn't. He used to ask what was wrong in a very aggressive way, and seemed to be suggesting that I was somehow deliberately withholding it for some reason. But he must have known from his own experience that sexual feelings are spontaneous and involuntary. So when I used to pretend, just to please him and stop him nagging me about it, he must have known that's what I was doing at least some of the time. Was it a kind of power game he was playing, forcing me to pretend? I wanted him to accept me as I really was, when I felt sexy and when I didn't, to respect my feelings.

When men pay a prostitute for sex they expect her to pretend to enjoy it, and maybe this feeling of power, of paying the piper, is the motive some husbands have in wanting their wives to pretend. When my ex-husband first suggested that I dressed up in fancy bra, suspender belt and black stockings it seemed like good fun, and I enjoyed it, but then he began to insist that I dressed for bed like that *every* night. Of course we didn't make love every night, but maybe he wanted to delude himself that I wanted him to every night. In the heat of summer it was very uncomfortable to wear stockings in bed and in the end I got totally pissed off with the whole thing. I suspected that these garments were becoming a fetish with him, that maybe he didn't need me inside them.

But I was glad to find that Dafydd wasn't like that. The dressing gown soon came off and we made love in a leisurely way, trying several different positions. He asked me what I enjoyed and I told him I liked being on top best. His favourite was doggie fashion. Everything we did was exciting, though. I was fascinated with his lithe, suntanned body. He looked so young and slim. He stayed all day and the following night, after phoning his parents to say he was staying with friends. The next time we made love it was in my bedroom, where I had a wall of mirror-fronted wardrobes. We stood in front of them for a while, undressing each other slowly and watching ourselves in the mirrors at the same time.

Dafydd's parents lived in a town about 20 miles away. He worked in London and was staying with them for the weekend, he said. So he had to go back to them on Sunday morning. He didn't give me their address or phone number, or his own in London. I felt regretful, yet in a way relieved. It had been a wonderful experience, but it was just sexual attraction and nothing else. For the first time I realised that I could have a casual affair without pretending to myself that I was in love, and without feeling guilty.

To my surprise he phoned me a couple of months later from London. It didn't feel right for him to have my number without giving me his. So I told him I had a new boyfriend and he didn't phone again.

After a while I thought it would be nice to have a proper boyfriend again, someone long term. I'd been afraid of emotional involvement, which was probably my subconscious motive for going around with Mair and Jade. Those two attracted one night stands like wasps to a jam jar. They were no longer on speaking terms with me since I'd 'pinched Mair's boyfriend' as they saw it.

I went out with quite a few men of various ages, but found that most of them bored or antagonized me on the first couple of dates. One or two I got on with really well in the social sense, but the physical attraction was lacking. This happened with a very good-looking man of 36 with whom I had a great deal in common. We went on long walks together, to the theatre, discussed novels we'd liked, cooked enjoyable meals at home for each other. But when he eventually tried to kiss me I just felt embarrassed. Perhaps we were so alike in our tastes that I felt as if we were too closely related.

And then there was Iolo, who really did turn me on. The sound of his rich, deep voice sent shivers down my back; his handsome face, his smile and the way he looked at me through his eyelashes had strange effects on my tummy: never mind butterflies, it felt like a whole aviary flying around in there. But he turned out to be a premature ejaculator. I'd never come across one before and never have since. I always used to think that if a bloke came too quickly it was because he was very excited and it would be better next time. It wasn't like that at all. I couldn't even touch him intimately – 'No, don't touch that, Melanie, it . . . whoops, too late!' and that was the second climax he'd had in less than an hour. There was one time when he succeeded in coming inside me and he was so thrilled he burst into hysterical laughter. But it had been so quick I hadn't had time to feel anything. He didn't seem to be much inclined towards any foreplay apart from kissing. He liked us both to lie naked and still next to each other. It was weird and I found it very frustrating. I had to tell him so after we'd tried on several occasions. I suggested he should seek professional help, but this really upset him so we agreed to call it a day. We got on well in every other way, and had a lot of interests in common. We also continued to see each other from time to time in the course of our work, so I'd hoped we could remain friends because I really liked him as a person. But on one occasion when we had lunch together (a couple of years after our brief affair) he asked if he could come round to my place that evening and 'make mad passionate love together, because it was so good before, I really don't understand why we parted.'

I stared at him in amazement and reminded him that we'd been sexually incompatible. He looked very sad and asked me why I said such hurtful things when they weren't true. Before we'd met his marriage had come to an end because his wife had gone off with someone else. Apparently they had both been virgins when they married, so it was obvious that she must have felt very puzzled and frustrated at the sexual side of their relationship, but he simply refused to admit that he had a problem. So our friendship had to end.

Another chap I went out with, Tom, was very big and quite ugly. He had ginger hair, pale freckly skin and had to wear thick bottle-bottom glasses because he was so shortsighted. When he took them off his eyelids looked pink and sore. But he was really good company, very witty and amusing. One winter's day we went on a long country walk in an area strange to us both, got lost and were benighted. Fortunately there was some starlight, although the new moon was hidden in cloud, as neither of us had torches. By the time we eventually found our way back to civilization I was beginning to feel very frightened. And the strange thing was that for the first time I felt sexual desire for this man. As soon as we were in the car we kissed and cuddled for a long time, then went back to his house and made love. He lived quite a long way away from me, so we arranged for him to come and stay at my house the following weekend. He had been before, but had stayed in the spare room. Mid-week I found a message on my phone saying he couldn't come. When I tried to phone him back, his phone had the line discontinued tone. I wrote, but he didn't reply.

About six weeks later I found, to my horror, that I'd caught pubic lice. I got something from the chemist which got rid of them, and also a book from the library, which told me they could not be transmitted except through intimate contact. So it must have been Tom. Before him it had been many months since I'd had sex with anyone, and there had been nobody since. Then I remembered his telling me just before we made love that he had been with a woman who was 'a bit of a dog' about six weeks before, that he'd gone for an AIDS test afterwards and that he was clear. Apparently if you bath or shower once or twice daily that gets rid of the lice but the eggs, or nits, remain. So it takes several weeks for them to build up to the level when so many hatch out in between showers that you become aware of the problem.

I guessed that Tom didn't realise that, and it was probably the reason he stopped seeing me. Perhaps he thinks to this day that he caught the crabs from me!

Soon after this I began going for long walks with Ieuan, a very shy colleague I'd known for years. He was around my age and had lived with his mother until she'd died recently. Nobody had ever seen him with a woman before and some people thought he might be gay. Others said his mother had been very bossy and disapproved of girlfriends. I enjoyed our conversations and we found we had a lot in common, though in some ways we were opposites: he was an extreme introvert and I'd always been fairly outgoing. He said he was only looking for platonic friendship. I said I was looking for a lover who could be a good friend as well, or perhaps the other way round. As time went on I began to feel very strongly attracted to him, but he never made a move although he seemed to enjoy my company. Remembering Tom, I decided to go for an Aids test just in case. Fortunately I was clear. That incident had really frightened and disgusted me so I felt relieved to be in the company of someone I felt safe with. Ieuan was kind and thoughtful in lots of little ways. After a while I realised that he was very inhibited. He couldn't even bring himself to stroke my cat, although I said she would like him to.

As months turned into a year the attraction between us became achingly strong. If he happened to touch my hand to help me over a stile I felt it like an electric shock. Once or twice I'd tried to kiss him. The first time he was so nervous and over eager, he head-butted me quite painfully. The second time he started, involuntarily wiped his mouth with his hand then looked very embarrassed. That really upset me and I nearly stopped seeing him. Then I thought I couldn't bear to lose his friendship. I phoned him and told him how I felt. He said he was very sorry he'd hurt me and didn't understand why he'd reacted like that. But he didn't say whether or not he was attracted to me sexually. I'd already asked him, in my forthright way, whether he was gay and he'd denied it instantly and emphatically. I decided to carry on just being friends and try to stop wanting more.

Eventually, inevitably, there was a one night stand with a very charming, glib womaniser called Jerry. He was an unqualified psychotherapist and I'd heard that he was in the habit of seducing his clients. I met him in a social capacity, but after inviting me in for coffee he sat me on the other side of his desk in his plush consulting room.

'Do you like playing doctors and nurses?' I asked coyly.

'Why, do you?'

'No, I thought perhaps you did.' He imagined he was seducing me, but really I just wanted a man to relieve my sexual frustration. He was an expert at kissing and foreplay. I lay back and enjoyed it. But this time I had some Durex in my handbag and insisted he use one. At first he was annoyed and argued about it. Then he agreed. He kept saying, 'Ok, I'll put it on in a minute.' Then he slipped into me when I no longer had enough will power to push him away. So really he tricked me. He wanted me to stay all night at his place, but when it was over I left and went home – after we'd had a little chat about his psychological problem with making long term relationships. And that was my last casual affair.

Ieuan and I are in our sixties now, having been married quite a few years. My cat and I moved into his delightful Edwardian home in a leafy suburb of the city and spruced it up a bit. He's quite happy about stroking cats and dogs these days. And the amazing thing is that he's the most satisfying lover I ever had. I forget where I read this adage: 'You can't make a sexy man good, but you can make a good man sexy.' It's the best advice a woman could have.

50s

'I placed segments of orange on the cushion and practiced serious kissing, while Sandy Shaw sang Girl Don't Come . . .'

The Twelve Trees

JILL TEAGUE

From as long ago as I learned to count, I have checked that the twelve trees on the mountain, across the valley from my parents' house, remained rooted on the skyline. They were special trees, the type that children draw to fit into the perfect gardens of the perfect houses in their pictures of perfect worlds – sturdy trees in a supportive clump, grouped in twos and threes – together yet separate. In summer their bright green leaves were soft and overlapped. They also represented something to me then – that a child doesn't really know but has assimilated by osmosis – of time and place, and of my position within both. They were strong and dependable – set apart but just in sight, temptingly, on the line where solid meets air, up and out of the rut of the valley.

In early childhood, despite my mother's most valiant efforts to feminise me with hair slides of all descriptions and yards of different ribbons for my hair, I remained refractory. I was unimpressed with the most up-to-date hand knits that she had spent hours after work fashioning for me. I particularly dreaded the arrival of spring, which inevitably led to my being bought a new poplin duster coat and a travesty of a bonnet with elastic under the chin. It took all of ten minutes for me to turn their delicate pastel shades to grey. This wasn't done out of malignancy on my part, it was just that the terrible burden – the disparity between how I looked and what I felt inside – became too much to bear. The role of little girl rejected me rather than the other way around.

In my primary school yard I tore around, inventing games and manufacturing situations where I could be the hero and rescue damsels in distress. My girlfriends followed me further up rock faces, and out across rivers, than sense or their own inclination would have taken them. But with my encouragement, they frequently found themselves out of their depth and in need of rescuing, and I relished each episode. I delighted in their screams and pleas for assistance, and the opportunity it provided for me to protect and comfort them.

Carol Edwards was by far my favourite. She stood at least six inches taller than me, and was, in fact, fairly robust. Nonetheless, at playtime, if she ever fell, got stung or into any other difficulty, a host of little kids would come to find me, and I gladly gave up any private adventure or challenge I might have set myself, to come to her assistance. It pained me to see her hurt in any way. We became inseparable as I cosseted her and lavished my time and energy on her. My desire was to see her happy and, maybe occasionally, to hold her hand or rest it momentarily against my cheek.

This intense relationship lasted a whole two years until her family moved a mile or so away onto a newly built housing estate. It wasn't the physical distance that separated us but the nature of the site. It was in a tougher area than our docile terraced streets were and when, a year later, the family emigrated to Australia, I grieved only a little, as I had already lost her to the rough boys.

At the start of the sixties I was eleven years old. My Uncle Ivor, refusing to follow his father and brothers down the pit, had made good as a builder. His relative affluence evidenced itself in 1962 with the purchase of a brand new Ford Zephyr Zodiac Mark III, in two-tone blue. John Glen was orbiting the world in a matter of hours, and my uncle was spending the same time taking the extended family, in carefully planned pecking order, for spins around the streets, up over the top of Trebanog Hill and back via the Colliers Arms. And while Rachel Carson was expressing concern for the race and planet regarding the squandering and overuse of fossil fuel, my uncle was revving like a demon and emitting carbon monoxide by the barrel load. To add to this hedonistic ostentation, one or other of his teenage daughters accompanied him on these trips – as accessories – to point out the various features of the interior, and to help the very young or the aged or those worse the wear for drink, in and out of the car.

What I remember of the outing wasn't the smell of new leather, or the walnut dashboard, or the enormous steering wheel – it was the sharing of the front seat with my cousin, Mair. Unhampered by safety laws and unencumbered by seat belts, I was sat on her lap so that the full contingent of the family on my Auntie Lily's side could crush into the back seat. At this time, Mair was a blossoming beauty of seventeen, wearing a button-through lambswool cardigan and a bell skirt, with her hair swept up into a beehive.

During the journey, my constant observations of her were made through the distortion of the windscreen and side window. The echo of her laughter rippled through me in gorgeous waves. But most of all, I remember the feel of her breasts, made unrelentingly prominent by her hard-cupped brassiere, in my back. It was for this reason alone that I wanted the journey to last forever. I sat as still as a preying reptile, feeling my tongue swelling from the lack of swallowing. Questions addressed to me went unanswered, and I could tell that my role as family idiot was in the making.

This excruciating blend of frustration and embarrassment culminated in a horrifying incident at the end of the journey. As I waited for Mair to dig out the last of the relatives, my gimlet eyes set on her arching back, I inadvertently slammed the door shut on Uncle Rhys's fingers. The air was blue with his shouting and swearing, cursing me – the family twp – in flourishing metaphors. Despite Mair's tender attempts to protect me from these verbal shafts, my pride was decimated, and I took myself off to pout in private.

After this, desire and guilt weaved like cross-wired skeins

throughout what was left of my childhood and adolescence. Whenever I recalled this early mortification, I went puce with shame, remembering, too, how closely pleasure is followed by pain.

Not long after this incident, my mother, father and I went on holiday, to stay with my mother's cousin, Dilys. Dilys had left the valleys a good few years before, taking her spouse from Stanleytown with her. They had set themselves up running a thriving transport café on the edge of Wimbledon. We were woken up regularly at five each morning as Dilys banged and clattered her numerous pots and pans. The air was a constant hazy blue from fry-ups and we weren't expected to be out any night after nine p.m. But all of this did nothing to dampen my ardour for Dilys's oldest daughter, Sian.

Sian Evans was a perfect blend of Cathy McGowan and Cilla Black – a stalwart Mod amidst the Rockers who frequented the café. She spoke with a slight lisp, had crooked front teeth and teenage acne, but to me she was perfection. For that short time in summer she showed me a wider world of stock car racing, fast food chains and the Kings Road. I was smitten. We shared a bedroom and I watched her undress each night, catching every possible angle in the triptych dressing table mirror. I counted the nights and days left to the end of the holiday with trepidation. The barb of my desire had embedded itself deeper this time, and I pined for weeks after returning from the holiday, playing and replaying Billy J Kramer's 'Bad To Me' on my powder blue Dansette record player, as Sian's short, dutiful letters to me dried up from a lack of interest on her part.

After that summer, I started at the local all-girls grammar school. My waking hours became a frenzy of infatuations and my sleeping ones awash with lurid, quasi-sexual dreams and nightmares. With an urge that I had no understanding of, I battered myself against the sharp edges of ridicule and rejection, swimming against the tide like a demented salmon.

I spent unduly long periods of time over the lingerie pages of catalogues, and in the dim living room light, I placed segments of orange on the cushion and practised serious kissing, while Sandy Shaw sang 'Girl Don't Come', barefoot.

However, I was to wait a further couple of years, watching my friends sprout breasts, paint their nails defiant red and date the most unsuitable of boys, feeling a traitor in their camp, before my first love presented herself to me. We shared a sense of humour, honing our sarcastic wit on each other. To outside observation this sparring was an obvious courtship, but we remained naïve. My bedroom was our bolt hole, with the gas fire baking half of each of our faces in winter, or the sash window down in summer letting in the manic street laughter of the kids we'd left to childhood. On Sundays we had brown bread and butter with tinned fruit. She always passed on the glace cherry to me, leaving its bled juice on the remainder of her own fruit.

We spent days out in the city or at the seaside, but always found ourselves back in my room. We lay in the dark with Stevie Wonder's voice cracking over 'Sylvia, you know you're getting to me now', our desire palpable.

It came as no surprise to me that when the time seemed right, I suggested we visit the twelve trees – somewhere we'd never been before. It was a day that burned with a light that holds open an autumn day and lets summer back in. The way was uphill and convoluted, and like our whole relationship, we did it without any points of reference. Climbing one tree, and looking back at my house and bedroom window, felt like making a journey from finish to start – all relevant markers looked strange. We were out on our own up there. I swung suspended from the branch and saw her eyes on the naked space of flesh where my sweater had risen up. Emboldened, I took her then into the ferns, half brittle with the changing season, and we kissed until our mouths hurt and were red rimmed. Then I touched her in every place that I'd ever wanted to on every girl or woman I'd ever desired, studiously ardent, until the sound that had lain embedded like a sliver of ice in my subconscious tore through the membrane of silence and melted us.

It was the coldness of the ground and a gathering darkness that stirred us for the walk home, holding hands in confirmation of each other and of our consummated love. We kept them that way until we reached the first of the houses, and, looked back then, to the last of the twelve trees soughing on the hill.

Sapphic Passions: from a Welsh Closet to London and Lesbian Lust

VRON GREGG

To the Irish nuns at my South Wales convent, the word SEX was highly emotive, with connotations of uncontrollable urges. A concept (let alone an act) regarded as only marginally less heinous than Communism. This, after all, was the 1950s, a time when the Cold War was very much at the forefront of people's minds. Marshall Tito, in the eyes of the Mother Superior, was the very incarnation of Evil. Aged 8 or 9, I knew nothing whatsoever about politics or the Eastern Bloc, but Sex . . . well, I'd garnered the odd snippet among my peers, and in the newspapers (albeit in less lurid terms than today). I was still at primary school, escaping – at 12 – the lengthier and more turgid lectures on carnal passions, but not before enduring the odd slobbery kiss on the cheek from music teacher Mother A, leaning over the piano with her bad breath and pent-up sapphic tendencies between my faltering arpeggios and the Angelus bell at noon. Everything, thankfully, stopped for the Angelus.

These were innocent times, when mothers could let their offspring roam the countryside freely, on bike or foot, without fear. Children in post-war Wales were relatively unsophisticated. The nuns lectured us girls on the importance of Good Manners, of maintaining a 'lady-like' demeanour at all times. No crossed legs, no trousers, and a ban on Boys, even in our heads. To think impure thoughts was in itself a sin. We inhabited a minefield of euphemisms in which nothing was

43

. The effect of all this of course
sity about sex and foster gossip
t wildly inaccurate.

I changed schools. I was 12 years
ral convent to secondary school in
eap, a massive culture shock. Instead
the bus stop, there was a regular free-
erly people were sworn at and shoved
asid for a seat. Sex was no longer a taboo topic.
Second-yea ls bragged about boyfriends to anyone who
would listen, and inhibitions floated away from me like layers
of clothing on a crowded beach.

My best friend Mandy and I went ballroom dancing on
Saturday nights at a club near the Uplands. It was a dancing
school where you could learn to do the waltz, quickstep,
foxtrot, tango and cha-cha. Some, like Mandy, went in for all
the medals as if born to it (a good mover was our Mandy).
Me, I took my bronze, just for a dare (I passed). But Saturday
night was open to everyone, a fun night out, with plenty of
slow dancing to scratchy 78s of Mantovani and Victor Silvester.
Rock'n'roll was the new religion and I took to it with all the
gusto of the freshly converted. It – and the club – were a
welcome escape from the doldrums of a town (Swansea had
yet to attain city status) which had endured more than its
quota of bombing. There was a grey, jaded feeling about the
town which dancing helped to dispel.

We jived to Elvis, Buddy Holly, Jerry Lee Lewis, Little
Richard, Connie Francis and the Everly Brothers. For me, the
music was the thing, the juke box the main draw. The male
clientele was a constant source of disappointment, consisting
mainly of macho, sweaty, gum-chewing Teddy boy clones
with string ties and sideburns and – in some cases – the most
appalling BO. I was 16 and two months when I had my first
proper kiss. Dave, who worked down the docks, was 19, short
and stocky with eyes like tiny dots glinting behind a pair of
thick, heavy-duty specs. Conversation was not his forte. We

went to the pictures a couple of times and indulged in some frenetic back-row necking. Then along came Mike, tall and gauche but a passably good dancer, followed by a few more 'insignificant others'. Until, one night, I met Eddie, a plumber, softly spoken with deep brown eyes. I was just 17. He was 25 (my parents were less than ecstatic about the age gap, and what they perceived as the class gap). Eddie and I were soon Going Steady. He was a fabulous kisser, which made up for his two-left-feet style of dancing. Mandy called him my 'bit of rough'.

Come the nine o'clock break, most of the blokes would head for the pub and come back reeking of stale booze and fags. Eddie and I would call in at Joe's ice cream parlour for a coffee, then he'd walk me home, along the Mumbles Road, stopping for a surreptitious snog in the sand dunes. On one occasion – big mistake – I asked him in. A tray of tea was produced, with a plate of Rich Tea biscuits, but the atmosphere was stony with parental disapproval. There were more pauses than words in our exchange. Afterwards, 'What's his father do?' Dad asked, as dads did in those patriarchal days.

I was very much the innocent abroad, uncertain precisely where the 'line' was drawn between Heavy Petting and Going All The Way. Once, after we'd both downed rather too many lagers, I was aware of Eddie's hand sliding up my leg, under my skirt and into my knickers. I woke the next morning, frozen with panic, recalling – but only hazily – the events of the night before. The rational Me knew that nothing had 'happened' and that I was still, technically, a virgin. But the over-imaginative Me wondered if I'd actually, inadvertently, Done It. Had I suffered an amnesiac lapse? Or was I simply too pissed to remember? Mandy, six months older than myself and a lot more experienced in such matters, was incredulous to the point of disdain. 'Don't be stupid. You'd know about it if you had. It usually hurts like hell the first time,' she scoffed as we strolled along the cliffs at Caswell Bay the following day, blowing away our hangovers. Sunday morning was post-mortem time: comparing experiences, slagging off last night's saddos, sharing adolescent angst.

In 1963 I left Wales to sample Swinging London. I was young, up for it, and my hormones were racing. I was looking for fun and freedom. I began exploring my sexuality, dating men to prove my heterosexual credentials while lusting after women, who usually (in those days) turned out – maddeningly – to be straight but who (I convinced myself) almost certainly had les/bi leanings. I never could resist the Unattainable, still can't. Too often, though, it ended in tears (mine). At first, like crushes on teachers (and I'd had a few of those), it was all strictly platonic, fear of rejection acting as a brake on my desires. I was far too scared to be open about how I felt, let alone make a pass. All the time I was being seduced by men, my thoughts would stray to the current Woman of my Dreams.

My first serious Crush was G, a work colleague. I was 20 and she was 28: plump, tactile and motherly, with an outrageously wacky wit. I adored her but, unhappily for me, she was very definitely a Man's Woman. She seduced me emotionally and broke my heart. We'd often socialise after work and lived under the same roof for a time, a situation engineered by me when I found out she was flat hunting. But we never did get to share a room, let alone a bed.

I only had eyes for G, my gaze rarely extending to my other three female flatmates. As far as I was concerned, they were invisible, a waste of space. Then along came 'Frank' and destroyed my idyll. He moved in and monopolised the kitchen with nightly fry-ups. He and G had a whirlwind romance, embarrassing us all with their public displays of snogging. I was in torment in the weeks before their wedding, trying to avoid G both at home and at work. She made the situation worse by going out of her way to include me in their social life. At night I resorted to earplugs, which failed to muffle the sounds of pre-nuptial euphoria from the other side of the wall. Masochistically, I accepted the invitation to their wedding. I'd had this fantasy where, at the bit in the wedding service about 'just cause or impediment', I would rise up from the organ loft and loudly proclaim to the congregation. 'I LOVE HER!' and 'DON'T DO IT!'. But when the actual, real-life moment came, I stayed in my seat, my lips well and truly zipped.

It took me months to recover. This, don't forget, was in the days before counselling became the accepted norm, recommended for just about every eventuality. Long before the arrival of any lesbian and gay helplines. I confided in no one and was in denial about my feelings for many months to come. It never occurred to me that I might be lesbian: role models at that time were limited and mostly of the butch-dyke variety and I thought, 'That's not me.'

I lay low for a bit before falling very heavily for B, another work colleague, at a job in publishing. We shared a tiny, window-less office off Berkeley Square, and often went out for lunch together. I was infatuated with her, so much so that she only had to brush against the back of my chair and I would sense the colour rising from my throat, through my cheeks and right up to the top of my forehead. My heart would pound away in my chest and I felt as if I was going to pass out. If B had any inkling at all of my inner feelings, she certainly never showed it. Meanwhile, my concentration waxed and waned as I dreamed the days away in a stupor of suppressed, unrequited lust.

Despite the freewheeling mood of the Sixties, options and outlets for lesbians and gays were depressingly limited, social acceptance was still aeons away, and the closet represented the only safe haven. So for a while I carried on dating men, courting male approval and popularity, passing for straight, pretending. I went through many months of two-timing liaisons in a desperate, last-ditch, attempt at showing the world I was 'normal'. A case of the lady protesting just a wee bit too much? Sexual activity, as I recall, was fairly low-key. Lots of kissing and cuddling. Fun without fucking. No intercourse as yet, (though I did try it with another guy later on, just for the experience, but found it to be fucking without fun). If challenged, I probably would have denied, in my defence, having sex with any of them. Shades of Bill Clinton when he denied having 'sexual relations' with Monica Lewinsky, thus triggering a sniggering debate about semantics.

One man I'd been 'seeing' wanted us to get engaged. I was briefly tempted, as JP was the kind of bloke – middle-class, unfailingly courteous, kind, intelligent, a newly qualified lawyer with Prospects – whom I could have brought home to Mum and Dad, amassing bucketfuls of brownie points and erasing all past transgressions at a stroke. We were well matched in terms of our interests (eclectic), temperaments and star signs (him Pisces, me Gemini). We enjoyed each other's company over wine-soaked meals in West End trattorias, conversing for hours about the Third World, literature, theatre, the meaning of the universe. There was just one snag: he didn't turn me on.

I was singing in an all-female pop group at the time: four of us were being groomed as a kind of quasi Ronettes, posing in flimsy femmy dresses for publicity photos in Trafalgar Square. The group turned out to be a useful get-out clause in our relationship: rather than admit to my preference for women (I was barely admitting it to myself, after all), I could proffer my musical aspirations as a handy excuse for declining JP's proposal of marriage. Having sat in on some of our rehearsals, the poor fellow could see for himself that music figured pretty high on my list of enthusiasms and he just couldn't compete. So we eventually parted. The group folded not long afterwards, in the wake of our one and only record release.

Everything changed when I answered an advert in a lesbian magazine, one of the few in existence in the late 1960s. That's how I met M, my first lesbian lover. My identity switched, overnight, from the role of tentative bisexual to that of eager-to-learn lesbian. At last I understood what all those soppy, Moon-and-June love songs were about. All my senses were heightened. It sounds corny, I know, but the sky seemed much brighter, colours richer and more vibrant, scents and aromas more pungent. Sex with M was sensational, sweeping all past and present male liaisons into the sidings of herstory. It was like waking up after a long lonely sleep.

Most weekends were reserved for M, who lived out of London. I don't remember too much of what we talked about as we spent nearly all our time in bed. M was an expert teacher, and I, at 23 years old, a quick and voracious learner. Sex, like singing, fast-forwarded the hours and I lost all track of time. I don't know what we did for food.

I can remember, after our first weekend together, travelling back on the District Line in a post-orgasmic daze to my bedsit in Fulham, my face bathed in a great big Cheshire-cat grin. I felt fantastic. Part of me longed to tell everyone I knew (and even some I didn't know), but coming out, then, was not an option. Despite the libertarian, anything-goes image of the sixties, heterosexuality was the norm throughout that decade. And so my sex life remained a well-kept secret (until the gay liberation movement changed the whole social climate in the early 1970s). A few months into my affair with M, the pressure of it all became too much. I was shattered, shagged-out, tired of juggling boy, girl, group, work. Something had to go – and it was JP. Like I said, I blamed it on the music. Poor JP. He'd have made a fantastic catch for some nice homely Welsh girl looking for a quiet, uncomplicated life. He deserved better than a crazy mixed-up, wannabe lesbian pop singer.

I'm sure that JP had no idea about my 'other' life. If I was in denial about being a lesbian, how could I expect others to know what I was up to? But I guess he must have had an inkling: he was, like most Pisceans, a sensitive soul, and my increasingly lukewarm response to his advances must have given him a clue.

Since then I've had two other long-term relationships with

women, plus two or three brief liaisons. I'm more grounded now, more comfortable with my sexuality. Age and perhaps a little wisdom have replaced the impetuosity of youth. And I've substituted writing for singing, although music will always be my first love. As for other passions, well, I've been celibate for a while now, but I'm open to more adventures when the time is right.

Indian Summer

ANON

I had no inkling of my true sexuality until I was in my late fifties. Certainly the possibility that I was multi-orgasmic had never occurred to me. By then I had been happily married for thirty years and had three children. I was a grandmother, for goodness sake!

There was passion in our early years of marriage, with a natural progression into warm, affectionate marital sex, not very frequent but nice when it happened. However, when my husband was in his early sixties, matters went incomprehensibly awry.

At first, when he was unable to achieve an erection, we tried to pretend it didn't matter. We even joked about it, in a strained kind of way. But of course it was in no way funny. He went to see our GP, a kindly man. Hard to tell who was the more embarrassed of the two.

His advice was to try injections of a drug whose name I have long since forgotten. It was, of course, before the advent of Viagra. My husband was told to inject himself immediately before intercourse.

Well, I ask you! Can YOU think of anything more off-putting? But we soon had far more worrying matters to deal with when my darling husband became terminally ill.

We went away for a last weekend together. Because of the nature of his illness he was scared even to attempt intercourse. Sex was off the agenda. It was scarcely even thought of during the ensuing months of battle – which he lost.

I had four years on my own – a life remade, with the help of loving family and friends. Work I loved, travel, one or two 'dates' arranged by well-meaning couples. One of the 'dates' made a clumsy pass. My gut reaction was "Ugh!" As far as I was concerned, that was that. In any case, I could not imagine that I would ever fancy another man.

Then, out of the blue, it happened. Never would I have believed myself capable of feeling such an overwhelming physical attraction.

From the moment I met this man, all I wanted was to go to bed with him. The sexual chemistry was overwhelming.

The sex was a revelation. He touched me so gently, so tenderly, with a kind of reverence, even, working down my body with kisses, his hands on my back, ever moving, ever caressing. He moved upwards, between my thighs. I was already soaking wet and ready for him. I put my hand on his penis. It was rock hard. He was ready, too. More than ready.

"It's been a long time, hasn't it?" he said, softly. Yet still he made me wait, holding me down, skilfully moving so that his erection was not in contact with my skin. Now he shifted his position, sliding down the bed until his head rested between my legs.

He licked tenderly, with tiny flickering movements of his tongue around the G-spot, probing deeper and deeper, bringing me to the brink yet not allowing me the final surge. Now, at last, he moved over me, to rub with his inflamed member the place where his tongue had so lately explored.

Then at last it was time. He slid into me. As I climaxed, he came with me, uttering small barking sounds, like a puppy. Damp with perspiration, we clung together, then rolled apart. But not for long. We had very little sleep that night.

You could say that I was starved of sex which, of course, I was, although without realising such to be the case. Neither had it dawned on me that I was one of those women fortunate enough to be multi-orgasmic.

The magic hasn't stopped, you see, even though we have

lived together for five years. Still, when we sit beside one another in the car, or the cinema, I quiver involuntarily. Sometimes, I glance at his crotch and look quickly away.

What causes such an overwhelming sexual attraction? Who knows? An excess of libido, perhaps. Now and again, my thoughts wander back to a coach trip we made during the long hot summer when we first met. We sat on the back seat, like a couple of teenagers. Only few teenagers would have dared to behave in such a way.

It was not just hands we held in that back seat. He took it out for me, you see. So big it was, and hard, moist at the tip, just the way I like it.

Then he put his hand beneath my skirt, sliding his fingers into the damp slithery wetness.

'You'll come quickly,' he whispered. And I did.

The Summer of Love

ANNE-RUTH ALTON

The Number 67 bus is now routed past Hosanna House on its way into town. Funny, because it was in 1967 that I was in there myself while all the world outside was going crazy with Flower Power. I sit forward, anxious to catch my first glimpse of 'The Loony Bin' in years.

As I do so the faces of the other patients swim into my mind: Shirley, Eleri and Glenys, Bryan, Hedwyn; Dr Lewis and Marianthe and the nurses. No doubt there were more, smaller fry in my imagination. Wondering what has become of all of them and whether I am the only one left to remember and record Hosanna House just as it was in the late '60s, I lose the present.

'People think that mental illness means the lack of a structure,' I once remarked, trying to impress a man, 'but that isn't so. Psychosis has its own patterns, as much as anything else does.'

First Uncle Rodney molested me between the ages of eight and ten and then, and all around it, was the bullying by my schoolfellows. 'Abuse', 'bullying' – those words were not so much on the agenda then and since I thought the fault lay within me, it did not even occur to me that they might have been what was happening. And if it had, I know that I would have been afraid to voice them even to myself. Certainly I could not speak of them to my parents or to Dr Lewis and Marianthe when they visited me at home when I was fifteen. And it was easier to stop striving when one was so unvalued.

'We've got a ward where we can look after you. Would you like to come?' Marianthe was so loving on that day, studying poor little me with her big dark eyes. She wasn't wearing one of her mini kaftans then, but within a few weeks of me being on the ward I became used to seeing this fifty-five-year-old woman in one most days, revealing herself in other ways too to be a totally contrasting person to the one she initially seemed to be.

I entered Hosanna House with a feeling somewhere between renunciation and relaxation. It was easier not to have to pretend that things were all right and I know I had a high awareness of my own drama. 'I'm only fifteen and I'm having a breakdown,' I thought, not unpleased with myself.

The Number 67 turns into the bus station – in my reverie I have missed seeing the hospital but, despite the events of the intervening years, I still feel the excitement of town. Boyfriends, the steel works, interesting shops, the fascination of working-class people, are its ingredients. Leaving the bus station, I turn left up the steep street. At the top I glimpse the plant and miss the smell of its pollution in the air. I remember the bright orange flare from the furnace touching up the night sky as I sat in the lounge with the curtains undrawn late at night in Hosanna House. I had just witnessed an act of sexual love.

On my first day there Glenys showed me around. She had long blonde hair and wore a red mini skirt. Soon I discovered that she had a different coloured mini skirt for each day of the week. She was an art student and was having a nervous breakdown due to a broken romance. She was slim and seven years older than me. At fifteen and twenty two, that is a huge gap and we never became friends, but I observed her as she seemed to me to epitomise the zeitgeist. Like others of my gods, she appeared hard but perhaps she was just trying to put me off.

On the evening I saw her making love, I had noticed her sitting between the open legs of a young man in the lounge on our ward. I was shocked at such a public expression of sexuality. One of the things I had tried to give up on entering the ward was touching myself – in private. It had never occurred to me to do it in public. I needed to like myself and I did not think that nice young girls masturbated. I cannot remember being aware of my own sexuality until Uncle Rodney introduced me to it. I hated him for it at the time. Pat, pat, pat he went with his big paw on my private parts; pat, pat, pat he made me go at the same time, with my small white hand on his old man's fly. How awful was the reciprocity of it! Once he unbuttoned himself (men of a certain age still were wearing button flies in those days) and forced my fingers inside. What I touched then, I thought of ever afterwards as a rod, because of his name and the stiffness of it and, by association, when I came into Hosanna House as a teenager and sat looking out of the window at midnight at the glow in the sky, the steel works reminded me of Uncle Rodney's rod. He died of a brain tumour when I was fourteen. When I worked on myself in the intervening years, I got a migraine.

In 1967, diagnosed with schizophrenia, I was aware of both my own innocence and taintedness and cast about in my mind amongst the other girls in my class at school, trying to guess which ones of them had also experienced sex, in one form or another . . . some of them had boyfriends already. I had not had a boyfriend yet.

The evening I saw Glenys having sex, I had gone to bed early. I had also practically given up eating because I was trying to make myself look more like Twiggy. Denial of my appetite left me with little energy and sometimes I felt exhausted. Although the sky could stay light as late as 10 pm it was dark when I woke. I could tell that through the chinks in the skimpy curtains in the women's dormitory. In the next bed to mine an older woman snored. I had come suddenly awake and was not, at first, sure what had woken me. Then I became aware of whispering in the bed opposite mine. There were six beds in the dormitory, two rows of three facing one another. Mine, and the one opposite me, were next to the door, so a little light came in from the landing. The Stelazine capsules I was taking could give you night-time blindness as a side effect, but I could still see the curve of two faces close to one another in that bed. It was Glenys's bed. At first I thought that the lad whom she'd been sitting with in the lounge earlier must have crept into our dormitory but then I became aware that the other voice was also female and that it was Shirley's. The remaining women in the dormitory seemed to be deeply asleep – most of them were on Mogadon.

Shirley was tall with short hair and full of experiences at the age of twenty. She had been working in London and 'grossing £100 a week' as she announced one day in the lounge. She was not pretty like Glenys, but she was more friendly towards me and had included me in some of the outings she arranged.

'Have you had it off with him?' she whispered angrily now.

I could not hear Glenys's reply.

'It's me you love,' continued Shirley, fiercely, and I heard the suck of lips on lips as, I guessed, her head came down over the other girl's. 'Me, me, me.'

Her vehemence reminded me of Cassius Clay mesmerising his opponents on televised boxing matches with 'I'm the greatest', as if by saying it, it became true. At that time I was telling myself that I was small and selfless, like my mother.

Shirley was panting loudly and I was afraid, for their sakes, that one of the others would waken and report them. When Uncle Rodney abused me in public places I was similarly afraid for him that other adults would catch him at it, my parents even, while at the same time I loathed what he was doing.

I sensed, rather than saw, that she was the dominant partner and when I heard her cry out into the night like an owl, I thought: How ugly. I wouldn't want to be like her. Glenys whimpered slightly. It was so faint that I might have missed it had my hearing not been very acute. It was a gentle, satisfied sound, a baby's after taking its fill from its mother's breast. Some extra-sensory perception made me see the smiling curve of her cheek as she rested her head on Shirley's shoulder in the bed and the pale, exciting down on her upper lip. Despite her acts and her clothes, Glenys's body and her bodily needs were somehow largely backgrounded but for that one feature – understated, refined. It was what I thought of as a 'quiet' body – you could not live closely to other women and not also have a sense of what their bodies stood for – and I aspired to the same *un*physical body as Glenys's.

No one else had woken. I lay awake in the dark, somehow satisfied because Glenys was. She and Shirley had fallen asleep and I wondered what would happen in the morning when the others woke, or when the ward sister came in and found them together in bed like that. I swung my feet onto the cold lino and stood up, almost tripping over the hem of the nightgown I'd borrowed from Eleri when my own pyjamas had got wet through a burst hot water bottle. (Eating little also made me feel cold, though the weather was warm.) I tip-toed out of the dormitory – I didn't want to disturb Glenys and Shirley, who were sleeping like babies, their heads together now, one blonde, one dark and cropped on the pillow – and went downstairs. A group of nurses sat in the half-lit lounge, in a semi-circle. Someone was laughing. They stopped talking as I came in.

'You're drowned in that nightie, Anne-Ruth,' said one and it sounded like an accusation rather than the compliment on my smallness I'd hoped for. 'What are you doing up at this time? I'll get you a Mogadon.' I had the impression that I was disturbing them though they were supposed to be here for us, the patients. Sitting by the window with the sticky cup of Horlicks she brought me, the tablet still in my palm, I waited until the nurses appeared to forget me again and became engrossed in their own social-nocturnal world before pulling back the curtains and gazing at the impression of the steel works and the orange flare against the night.

In Hosanna House we saw Dr Lewis and Marianthe once a week, unless there was a group therapy session. They sat in a little office and we took it in turns to go in. They were contrasting individuals, Dr Lewis quiet and still in a dark suit, 'introverted' as we on the ward had decided when it occurred to us to reverse our roles and 'analyse' the psychiatrist. In fact, Marianthe was not qualified in that field. She came from Australia where she had been a gynaecologist and some of the older patients speculated that her unconventional methods had got her the sack. The story put about by the hospital authorities was that she was having a career change late in life. It seemed odd, but then Marianthe was unusual.

Like her eyes, her hair was dark and, as mentioned, she favoured mini kaftans, brightly-coloured, and large, dangly earrings except when she was visiting patients in their homes. Perhaps she wished to appear reassuringly 'normal' to the distressed families of the mentally ill. To wear those clothes at her age, a woman needed a good figure, and Marianthe was blessed with one. Her bone structure was elegant, her skin olive. I remember sitting in the office, not paying attention to whatever she and I and Dr Lewis were discussing, but instead observing her high cheek bones and connecting them in my mind to her slim, well-shaped legs and wondering how artificial she had to be to achieve her total effect, since I felt that, in this life, I could never be wholly who I wanted to be – inside or out – and could only approximate to an impression of smallness and *un*physicality by going to great lengths. Such as I was now by starving myself.

'Sister says you've gone under eight stone. Given your frame that's too low,' Dr Lewis was saying.

'Does the idea of having no energy and being a permanent

invalid appeal to you?' Marianthe asked. 'It does to some people.'

I sat in stony silence. This was not going a bit the way I wanted it to.

'You wouldn't have to make any effort then, little would be expected of you.'

Dr Lewis puffed on a Woodbine. His desk was arranged very precisely and every week, when I went in, his leather driving gloves were in the same position on it. I wondered if the arrangement was some kind of test so that he could tell how observant or otherwise we patients were.

'If you started to eat properly you needn't be in here much longer,' he commented.

'But perhaps you don't want to leave,' added Marianthe.

That was right. I didn't. I had never told them about Uncle Rodney or the bullying at school – it would have disturbed my self-image too much to admit to these things. And so they were left to speculate on why they had found me at home as they had, in the late spring, not speaking, uninterested, dis-engaged with life.

'You are a lot better since you've been on the Stelazine,' Dr Lewis told me.

I had not noticed this myself and was uninclined to accept it.

'Do you masturbate?' enquired Marianthe abruptly.

A blush was my reply.

'Why don't you get a boyfriend and have sex properly? It's only convention that prevents people.'

Mum said that boys wouldn't respect you if you let them and that if you 'had' to get married it would always be something you might blame one another for when things went wrong. I believed Mum and there was something else, something to do with not being able to let go, a barrier to 'going the whole way'. Of course, I did not express these thoughts to Marianthe. In any case, I wouldn't have been capable of formulating them so precisely then. My life has been a process of coming towards myself, Anne-Ruth with the large frame, Anne-Ruth who is very self-interested and quite physical.

Why were we talking about sex, I wondered; what had it got to do with me being here? (I did not count Uncle Rodney as a legitimate player in 1960's sexuality and his 'interference' with me had ended when his illness started in 1962. Again the image was wrong.)

I left the session with my head swimming, trying to gather my safe, pretty images together so that, as soon as I had crossed the corridor and returned to the semi-circle in the lounge, I would appear to the others to be the nice little girl with her Peter Pan collars I projected and whom they grat-ifyingly saw me as.

But, since Eleri was at the door, I could not immediately re-enter the lounge. Eleri was in her forties with frizzy black hair. She was large but still had a withered look. A man and two teenagers sometimes visited her on the ward. Every movement she made was slow, like an action re-play on television. Getting through a doorway took her between five and ten minutes on average. Perhaps she feared what she might find on the other side. I did not know what her illness was but it complemented mine in that I was able to add to my ideal of selflessness by undressing her and tucking her up in bed every night and making myself kiss her. She went to bed early. When it was her period she refused to wear any sanitary protection and, as I removed her blood-stained knickers, she would observe my revulsion and smile as if to say, 'You're not the saint you claim to be.' She always waited for me to kiss her once I'd accustomed her to it, but she never said a word. There were a number of people on the ward who either could not or would not talk about their illnesses. I did not know what was wrong with Shirley. Or Bryan.

Having gained the sanctuary of the lounge I sat down next to him. 'Hello,' he said. 'Hello.' For a while we sat in compan-ionable silence. He was seventeen, dressed very soberly and his whole aura suggested the previous decade – minus its Teddy boys. He liked Cliff Richard and The Shadows and spoke respectfully to people older than himself. He had sandy hair and a thin, taut, freckled face. He worked as a trainee printer on the local newspaper. He challenged nothing and no one.

'Why do you align yourself with Bryan? He won't make any demands on you,' Marianthe asked me.

'On your intelligence,' Dr Lewis added.

But Bryan was exactly what I wanted. We rested in one another. For him I adopted a jaunty 'with it' persona and imagined that I must be his Glenys. But as we sat in the lounge after the interview with the consultants that I have described, he suddenly said, 'Don't change as you get older, Anne-Ruth. You're a nice girl – not like them.' He nodded across to Shirley and Glenys, who were sitting holding hands opposite. They were making no secret of their romance, but so far no one else had seen them sharing Glenys's bed. Shirley must have had a built-in alarm which made her wake up in time to sneak back into her own before any of the older women in our dormitory had woken. And the two girls roused nobody except me with their midnight loving.

Once they stopped in mid-act and looked across at me, aware, it appeared, that I was watching them. In the darkness they could not, of course, be sure, but despite the Stelazine, I seemed to have X-ray eyes – or was it ESP? – as I felt them glance at one another before continuing with their lovemaking. They didn't seem to mind me knowing and I didn't feel like a voyeur. Their romance, now passionate, now gentle, brought a kind of peace into my life, probably because I felt that if this could go on and present a Swinging Sixties image then there was nothing about me – my well-developed bosom, my short legs, about which girls at school taunted me – that was truly unacceptable and which I myself could not eventually grow used to. Keeping this vigil in the women's dormitory at Hosanna House, I felt like some benign nightbird or divinity guarding over them lest anyone else awoke. But on it went, night after night, while Eleri and the other middle-aged women in the dormitory muttered in their sleep or snored. Myself, I was attracted to the opposite sex, some of the male nurses, the lad whose legs Glenys had sat between on the floor, a boy at school I sometimes dreamed of.

Bryan did not excite me and I'm sure he was aware of it. One day, after a lunch which I as usual did not eat and he, though thin, tucked into, we set out to walk around the hospital grounds. The sunshine was warm and the well-tended flowerbeds bright with blooms. The hospital had been a Victorian workhouse and, as we paraded past the redbrick villas of other wards, we could see looming in the centre the old clock tower. It was 2.15pm. We were talking about these other wards, some of which, in 1967,were still designated 'mentally subnormal' when Bryan asked, 'Do you think I'm normal?'

'What's normal?'

'You know,' he shrugged, 'go out to work, not like these hippies, get on with the blokes, go down the local at week-ends.'

'Do you ever dream, Bryan?'

'Eh?'

'Do you ever imagine that you are special and might be famous one day?'

He laughed. He was wearing a brown check shirt and had taken off his jacket because of the heat. He had a tie on. I could see that he didn't share my dreams.

'D'you fancy going to see Michael Caine in *Alfie* – it's on in town – if Dr Lewis will permit us?' he enquired.

Dr Lewis didn't object. In the cinema I sat with the box of Cadbury's Milk Tray Bryan bought me on my lap, not eating them (I passed them on to Eleri), and we giggled when the famous commercial came on the screen: a dare-devil man in a catsuit scaling perilous heights and walls and then, as he arrived in the lady's bedroom, the voice-over: 'And all because the lady loves Milk Tray.'

'He should have brought her to the Roxy and called in the sweets kiosk – it'd have saved him all that palaver,' whispered Bryan.

We sat, not touching, and not really engaging with the film. I found Alfie a selfish character and when we came out and stood at the bus stop, waiting to return to Hosanna House, Bryan said, 'That's what I mean. You don't meet blokes like that in everyday life. He's not normal, is he?'

A few days later when most of us were sitting in the semi-circle of chairs on the ward, we heard the shattering of glass from the men's dormitory above and saw, through the window, a wooden bedside locker come hurtling down to the ground. It was just like the pop song, 'They're coming to take me away, ha ha, they're coming to take me away' and two men in white coats did appear and did take Bryan, who was responsible for the incident, away.

That left me with Hedwyn to sit next to in the semi-circle in the lounge. If people were like animals then he was a bear, with the sometime cuddliness of a teddy and also the aggressiveness of a wild grizzly whose perceived source of provocation you could not guess at. His appearance too, was bear-like: big and bulky – he could not be dressed to look neat – with a shambling walk and loose joints. But Hedwyn was very straightforward and called a spade a spade and for this I became fond of him.

I suppose he was about sixty in 1967. He was a Roman Catholic and what had brought this great man down, brought him into Hosanna House, was the death of his dog. He showed me photographs of a wiry mongrel named Bingo and said, 'He was my best friend.'

'I think I prefer animals to people,' I remarked, trying the thought out for size.

Hedwyn peered at me through his short-sighted brown eyes. 'You're very young to be a misanthrope,' he commented.

Since I did not understand 'misanthrope' I did not reply.

'What's made you like that?'

I looked down, unwilling to meet the sincerity in his eyes. I felt again that my reasons for being here were not genuine.

The TV was on and showing young people sitting on the pavement in Haight-Ashbury with flowers in their hair. Like Glenys had done, some of the girls were sitting between the boys' open legs.

'Bloody permissive age,' growled Hedwyn. 'If it wasn't for your politicians, Roy Jenkins . . .' His resentment of the era was a byword. 'GPs handing out prescriptions for The Pill to young girls at the drop of a hat, respect gone out the door – you can't go in a shop and get SERVICE . . .' On he rabbited, until Shirley, who was sitting on his other side, and whom I did not think had been listening, abruptly turned round and tweaked his ear. 'Dinosaur,' she teased him.

He flushed with anger and, for a moment, I thought there would be a nasty scene, but suddenly all the forcefulness left him and he turned away from her and sat leaning forward, elbows on knees, looking sapped. It was sad to witness and also, for the first time, made me pay attention to what he had been saying.

If the circumstances arose, would I go on The Pill? Or did I believe what his religion and also the religion of my own father – who was a lapsed Catholic – taught about sexual morality? It struck me that I did not know what I might think or do five minutes from now. I was like a stalk blowing in the wind, subject to every change of direction.

In fact, my favourite pop group, The Animals, cashing in rather late on the turn of world events, had brought out a new LP titled 'Winds of Change' and, on my birthday, my parents brought it for me into Hosanna House. Shirley decided to throw a party on the ward, ostensibly in my honour, but I think she was just in the party mood.

I sat next to Eleri on a couch. She was still finishing off the box of Milk Tray and it upset me to think that with this 'gift' she had finally accepted me as a good girl and I was really betraying her trust by being more concerned with my self-image than with her wellbeing. I tried to visualise what Hedwyn might say if he could read my mind and I settled on a past comment of his whose connection was forgotten: 'Our Lady teaches us that by being false we diminish ourselves more than anyone: look how she responded to the news that she was with child, true to God and true to her own destiny.' Sitting next to Eleri, my eyes filled with tears.

Dr Lewis and Marianthe were dancing together, as best they could to the track *Hotel Hell* with its haunting trumpet solo and Eric Burden's deep plaintive voice singing 'I'm so very far from my home.' Dr Lewis's hands seemed to have found a home resting on the gynaecologist's bottom as the couple moved slowly across the carpet. He wore one of his dark suits and Marianthe a truly gorgeous evening dress: long jewel-encrusted, with a very deep V back. Perhaps her seat was a more innocuous place for his hands than her bare back, but I noticed some of the others watching them.

Suddenly I couldn't stand it a moment longer, got up, walked across to them and tapped Dr Lewis on the arm:

'Excuse me,' I said, 'will you give Eleri this dance?' He stared at me and I felt, without meeting her eyes, that Marianthe was studying me with amusement. However, he acceded to my request and went over to Eleri who got up with amazing alacrity.

Over Marianthe's shoulders, I could see the lad whose legs Glenys had sat between. He had long brown hair and wore denims. I could not see much of his face and knew nothing about him, but decided I was attracted enough and he would do. As usual he was sitting on the floor, his legs open. I went and sat between them. He said nothing and, after a few minutes, it occurred to me that he was probably a junkie and probably had not noticed the difference between Glenys deserting him for Shirley a few weeks ago and me taking her place.

When everyone appeared to be involved with someone

else at my party, we went upstairs to the dormitory and did it in my bed. We had taken no precautions but there was no unwanted after-effect.

When I returned to school in the new term, I felt so much older than my ridiculous schoolfellows, with their beliefs that this world, the world of smoking in the bogs and who was going out with who and which teacher was the nuttiest was the only world of significance. During the summer I learnt about different kinds of love: between Shirley and Glenys; the friendship I'd had with Bryan whom I visited on his new ward and who might have been 'possible' for me if he hadn't become so listless and who had one day commented: 'You're too good for me, Anne-Ruth'; a real affection I developed for Eleri; the safe-and-scared feeling I had with Hedwyn (scared when he capitulated); and the 'Kind of Loving'[1] with the junkie who, even in his drugged stupor, seemed to realise I was a virgin, and was quite gentle with me. I never did discover his name.

I walk up to the fence surrounding the steel works, which are now closed and I try to imagine what went on inside the plant at the height of its production. The connecting metal pipes in front of me make a geometric pattern and I picture men inside the plant running about with red-hot rods – doubtless an inaccurate vision. Could Uncle Rodney's rod be called red-hot? Years after The Summer of Love in Hosanna House, a friendly nurse said to me: 'Was he a funny old man? I had an uncle a bit like that. I told my Mum.' Although the plant has shut now, I can close my eyes and see a snug orange glow in my mind's eye, remembering those nights I sat up on the ward with the lounge curtains open, deciding who I was going to be.

---

1. 'A Kind of Loving' is a novel by Stan Barstow.

Nice Girls Didn't

RUTH JOSEPH

I am fifty-five. My married daughter would be disgusted that I am writing this story. But sex has been such an integral part of my life, as crucial as a limb or vital organ, that I cannot imagine it as shameful. It has played a major role in our lives, quite apart from the procreation of our children.

I was a child of the sixties when nice girls didn't. But there were parties and boys and a million hormones coursing round the darkened pillowed evenings when mouths and lips searched impatiently and eager fingers wandered through the forbidden territories of Crimplene and nylon. But nobody special for me.

My parents wouldn't let me go to get-togethers unaccompanied, so I enlisted a squad of young men happy to escort me. I was bigger then, twelve and a half stone, but rapidly lost two and a half stone on cranky diets. And I was hungry. Hungry to be the one wanted, *fancied*, longing to have a real boyfriend rather than the film star guys whose pictures postered my room. And I had fun and necked but that was that. The young lads touched my breasts but we never . . . I never . . . nice girls didn't.

Until I met my future husband. He rescued me on a bad night when a b . . .d, the chairman of our charity group, dumped me for another girl after asking me to be his special date. I discovered later that he wanted me for my cooking ability – someone to cook the salmons for the next day's party.

There I was, in an empty youth club building, crying tears

that echoed down the lonely concrete corridors, blubbing into two large fish kettles and two very dead fish staring red-eyed at my gold lame mini dress with a keyhole and my gold shoes.

Eventually, someone remembered me – very late – and I returned to the party. I smelt of a mixture of my mother's perfume and fish water.

He was standing in the shadows. I looked at him: slim build, a little taller than me. His eyes were kind. Large dark pools with the most ridiculous eyelashes for a man. He moved towards me.

'Can I get you a drink?' I said, acting as Charity Vice-Chairman and trying to pretend that I still looked . . . smelt . . . attractive.

'I think I should get you one,' he said.

'Mmm, Coke would be lovely.'

In seconds he was back. We talked and then we were dancing, the Rolling Stones, the Beatles and Motown rhythms pulsing, as our eyes ate hungrily. He pulled me closer and kissed me and I tasted the blackcurrant on his mouth. His lips were gentle and enquiring and for the first time something within me began to respond. He drove me home in a small maroon Mini. Under the shadow of the pine tree that hid the streetlight's gaze, his fingers travelled through layers of clothing. Finally we pulled apart but only because of my father's strict curfew which was twelve o'clock for a very special party.

'Come out with me tomorrow? Please? I'll ring,' he whispered.

I flew into the house to meet my invalid mother's scrutiny. My father had retired to bed and left her as timekeeper.

'You've been got at!' she said disgust colouring her voice. 'Look at your hair and your mouth!'

She was right, the beehive endowed with many layers of concentrated backcombing was no more!

'He's asked me out again tomorrow night,' I said tri-

umphantly, casually trying to tuck the stray curls into some
form of respectability.

I knew she wanted me to make tea – tell her about the
evening. But I wanted to keep it sealed tight in the party
wrappings of my mind. I made an excuse.

'I'll get you to bed.'

'No no, I'll manage . . . I'm not ready yet.'

I heard the unspoken sighs. I felt guilty. The first clash –
the first time a man's needs in place of my mother's wants.

I don't remember washing or getting into bed but I do
remember lying in my room – sixties yellow and black –
reliving his eyes and the way they crinkled with easy laughter,
his mouth and his slim fingers.

The hands on my watch limped as I counted the minutes
till eight the following night. I was happy. He made me laugh.
It was as if we had always known each other.

But I wouldn't go in the back of his Mini. Nice girls didn't.

Finally, three years later, we became engaged. And I agreed
to sleep with him. We were going to London to the Furniture
exhibition at Olympia with money from his father to spend
on our new home. My parents arranged for me to stay with
my aunt three miles away from my fiancée's hotel, so that
there would be no hanky panky. But she was a disinterested
jailer and let me come and go as I pleased.

It was a dark November afternoon when the day decided
to finish early. I was in his anonymous hotel room – terrified!
But his hands were slow and gradually he peeled my
London–grimed clothes from my body. We crawled into bed
and when he entered me, I didn't dip into a thousand stars.
We were awkward. I was tense, nervous, and neither of us
had any experience. I was nineteen. He was twenty-seven.
Wouldn't the young laugh today? After, I sat in front of the
dressing-table mirror looking at myself. I was amazed I
looked the same – surely there would be a change – I must
look different. The whole thing was a painful, sticky affair and

I bled for days. Now, as my mother accused on our first meeting, *I was got at.* I never told him it was painful. I just knew it would get better. It did.

Now we have been married almost thirty-three years. We know each other's bodies. He knows now that I take a long time to become aroused. It won't happen if the radio or television is on. I enjoy quiet. I want to concentrate on the feel and the scent of his cool male skin, reach up and touch the hair at the back of his neck – now white. I need him to speak sometimes but he finds this difficult. But when we are together, totally as one, we feel good – like the pieces of the jigsaw are linked to make the whole.

Sometimes we make love outside. We have moored on the side of the Abergavenny Canal and slept on a soft blanket in a dark forest, with the waters lapping close and the shrill cries of birds resonating in our ears. We have loved each other on the top of the Brecon Beacons with the sounds of sheep and cattle systematically munching around us. And once we made love on the top of Beachy Head in the black velvet dark, with the seawater smashing and sucking at the cliffs below. We must have been very good because that part of the cliff has now disintegrated and fallen into the sea.

Sometimes we indulge our fantasies. But usually only when we are on holiday. They take time. And we both like to plan the moment. Build up the excitement inside. Maybe after supper: a bowl of good pasta, a glass of wine, and some warm ripe peaches, we'll slip away from bright conversation, to the fairy light reflections rippling pianissimo on the lake. With his arm around me or hand in hand, we'll walk – a gentle evening's walk. He'll lean over and whisper to me that he wants to undress me slowly in a lit window. I used to worry about it but I don't anymore. Or he may ask me to go without underwear or just stockings and suspenders under a fitted dress.

'Will you do it for me tomorrow and wear your proper high heels?'

I know then to take a special bath before supper – plenty of fragrant oils and perfumed moisturiser which I never usually use. That evening, feelings become more exciting. Every touch burns with anticipation. But we linger. We watch the sun set in a million glittering diamonds on the burnished water. We have a small fruit ice cream taking a lick from each other's cone. We eat supper late, watching each other's eyes, pleasuring the conversation, touching fingers across the table. And then, after, the moment is perfect – explosive.

My fantasies are different. They take more planning but to me are special. They usually follow a hot afternoon and a cool rest when I have given my husband an all-over body massage. Then it is time to ask him. I lean over his body, kiss his closed eyes and those amazing eyelashes and ask him to make a date. I hanker to be laid on a mass of pillows, tied up with silk scarves, the room soft with candlelight, massaged with rose and orange-blossom oils, and his firm tongue on my skin. In my imagination, he is a prince or a gentle captor.

Our bodies are rehearsed and we can make love on a wet afternoon for hours, softly rubbing and licking; or, during a sultry siesta our passion can be noisy, wild and Technicolor, accompanied by the ticking of Mediterranean cicadas like a thousand impatient clocks.

There is no better way of sharing. I am fortunate. Most of my friends abdicated from the role of lover before the menopause. When we are away I am his mistress; when we are at home – his wife. Both are perfect roles. My daughter and son would be shocked that I have written this. Sex is the privilege of the young, they think. To them we are Mum and Dad: me hitting the henna bottle and him the grey-haired wise one who always gives good advice. But I never see him like that. When I look at him, the years have faded. We are back dancing on that first night, his soft brown eyes edged with those ridiculous lashes, his slim hands touching mine. The time when I wouldn't climb in the back of his purple Mini . . . when nice girls didn't.

This Voyage

ANON

I was twenty-five and three months pregnant the first time I masturbated. It was nineteen seventy-two and I had been married for three years. It was my first orgasm. I remember the guilt I felt afterwards, the disgust with myself. I had read an article in a magazine about a woman who had never climaxed with her husband through sexual intercourse. I didn't know what 'climaxed' meant, but there was a vague description of how she had masturbated and so I pressed my fingers between my legs. The harder I pressed the more overwhelming the sensation that something was happening. The force of the orgasm shocked me; I remember the muscles in my lower abdomen tightened spasmodically and I was horrified. And frightened that I'd damaged the baby.

Exhilarated yet ashamed, I vowed it was something I would never do again. Of course I did. I have never told my husband that I masturbate and I have always experienced guilt. The revelation of that orgasm made me recognise what I was striving for when we made love. John was my first boyfriend; we were both virgins when we married. He came from a very religious family and he has often said he never saw his mother and father kiss or even touch one another. And it was ironic that my first masturbation was during a weekend visit to my parents' house, because I also grew up in a household where sex was never mentioned.

Yet there are sexual memories. Standing outside the chemist's in town while my mother went inside to buy 'personal things'. The packet of Durex carelessly thrown onto their bedside table, its purpose questioned but unexplained. Seeing my mother in bed powdering her face and putting on make up, waiting for my father. Going to the lavatory in the morning and seeing a long pale translucent object in the water and being frightened.

More personally, I remember the feel of my father's warm arm between my legs as he came behind me and tipped me up and over the chair 'in fun' and the feel of his penis as he lay on top of me 'playing' at wrestling. I was eleven maybe twelve at that time and the sensation of his flaccid penis hardening against my body scared me, even though I didn't understand what was happening. When I tried to talk to my mother about it, she declared that my father loved me and would do nothing to hurt me. Which worried me even more as I had always presumed my parents loved me even if it was never said.

When I started to menstruate at thirteen I knew nothing, except for the whisper of dirty jokes that I had overheard on the school bus, and was shocked. That morning, as the pain rolled around inside me, my mother produced a sanitary towel with two loops at the end and a piece of elastic. Her short embarrassed demonstration indicated the way I had to thread the elastic through the loops and wear the thick wad of gauze and cotton wool, and I was sent off to school. She hadn't told me how to fasten the elastic so I knotted it to make sure it was safe. As the day progressed, each time I changed the towel I had to break the elastic which consequently got tighter and tighter around my waist. I can recall the pain of that now.

My mother must have told my father about my periods, because the wrestling stopped. However, as I developed, he joked about my breasts and often flicked at them with his thumb and forefinger. My mother wore the cone-shaped Playtex bras and he would take great delight in poking her breasts so that the bra dented in. He obviously presumed he was entitled to do similar things to me; it was humiliating. I became self–conscious, ashamed of my body. In stark contrast I can recall the occasion when, in my mid-teens, I announced that my friend's mother was pregnant. My father walked out of the room and didn't speak to me for a week. I was told by my mother that 'pregnant' was not a nice word.

There was another event that for years I refused to acknowledge as sexual. It happened when I was about ten. It was school holidays and our parents were both working. My sister, Katherine, told me we were going to play mummies and babies. I didn't know what to expect but was excited that she wanted to spend time with me. At fifteen she had a set of friends that didn't include me; I was probably a great nuisance factor in her social life. When she shouted for me to come into her bedroom Elvis Presley was singing on the radio and the curtains were drawn. Katherine was lying on the bed naked, her head resting on one arm and I remember her figure: pale skin, rounded breasts. I had never seen anyone naked before. She had hair around her pubic area, dark, curly. She told me to lie alongside her. I refused, saying it was a stupid game, but she retorted that she would tell Dad that I had asked her about the funny noises that sometimes came from their bedroom. This terrified me; my father was short tempered and often chastised us with his fists. She ordered me to suck her nipples. 'You're my baby.' I remember the firmness of her breasts against my nose; it was suffocating. Her skin was cool but damp. 'Play with me down there,' she said. I didn't know what to do. I recall feeling silly and uncomfortable. I got off the bed and ran downstairs. Katherine threatened to say it was my idea if I mentioned it; all I wanted to do was to forget the whole thing. Even now I have never told my mother. Around that time I had wanted to ask my sister if our dad 'wrestled' with her. After that afternoon I couldn't. As we got older we grew apart. My sister and I don't speak any more.

As we grew up there was always a comparison between

Katherine and me; she was everything I wanted to be: pretty, clever, confident. I was very jealous. Plump and plain, I hid behind thick National Health glasses. I struggled with school-work and I had few friends; certainly none of them were boys. Despite all this I still had secret crushes on some of the boys in the village. One in particular, Roy, changed girlfriends often. A favourite place for the youth of the village to congregate was the cricket club. Roy and his current partner would disappear round the back of the clubhouse. When they reappeared the girl was always flushed and dishevelled; he always swaggered. The rest of the group cheered and catcalled. Tolerated, as long as I didn't draw attention to myself, I would watch, desperate to belong to the group of girls who had 'been with Roy'. Whatever that meant!

When my dream came true I was sixteen and it was a wet Saturday afternoon in winter. Coming back from the shop with the bottle of milk my mother had asked me to buy, I passed the cricket field. There he was, sitting alone, smoking a cigarette on the pavilion steps. I remember the off-hand way he called me over to him; the way my heart thumped, thinking that at last he had noticed me. He held my hand as he took the milk and, putting it on the step, led me down the side of the clubhouse. As I closed my eyes and lifted my face to be kissed I was slammed against the wall of the building. There was pain in my head and I couldn't breathe. I was aware that he was holding me back with his shoulders, his head so tight against mine that my neck was twisted to one side and he was pulling at my jeans. This was one time I was glad to be fat; they were so tight around the waist it was impossible to undo the button. I have never forgotten that intense feeling of panic and fear. Although the details of those few minutes are confused I can recall the foul language, the pain as Roy grabbed my breasts, jammed his knee into my crutch and the way he rubbed up against me until he shuddered and stopped. In the fight, because that is how I most remember it, I had lost my glasses and, even though I was so short sighted that everything was a blur, I ran in the direction of home. I forgot the milk. I have no recollection of the aftermath of that day. I don't remember getting into trouble about either my glasses or the milk, or being later back than expected. Perhaps there was no one in when I got home. I don't know. I do know I have never told anyone before.

Initially, I was not going to write about that afternoon as there are many experiences more horrific suffered by other women and I felt it to be too trivial, but I have cried as I have relived that experience and all those old feelings of self-disgust descend on me. I feel it was yet another incident I allowed to happen and I realise how much that afternoon affected me.

By the time I was eighteen I had already left school, lost two stone and won my battle of perseverance with the old fashioned kind of hard contact lens. I went into the Civil Service and suddenly found I was attractive to the men I worked with. For the first time I had some power in a part of my life. Following my instincts I learned who to trust and how to flirt with the men I felt safe with, how to ward off any unwanted attention. But this was only in the office; I had no social life. My father had become increasingly moody over the years, as I grew more independent. There were many rows when he would shout, demanding to know who I had spoken to outside. 'It's not you I don't trust, it's those buggers out there!' he would declare, standing in front of the door and dragging out the quarrel until it was either too late to go out or just easier for me to stay at home.

One Monday morning I went into work to find there was a new face in the office. A face I thought was extremely handsome. It was John. I was very wary of him; in my experience good-looking boys were dangerous. But he was quiet, shy, and eventually, over some months, we became friends.

Before our marriage, engaged and feeling safe in my future
with John, though our sexual knowledge had progressed no
further than petting, I was less afraid of my father. Often he
studiously refused to speak to me, so at least there were no
arguments. But the atmosphere had a latent volatility; my
father was extremely temperamental, and I was relieved
when, after three years, John and I were quietly married in a
Register Office. Now, I can smile when I think of how sophisticated I thought I was, with my Mary Quant hairstyle, mini
skirt, long boots, pan-stick makeup and white lipstick.
However my self-confidence was a façade that hid a naiveté.
For our honeymoon we stayed for two nights in a local hotel.
On that first evening we sat in the bar trying to make the
drinks and conversation last as long as possible. Eventually
John suggested that we go to our room. I remember shaking
as I put on the nightdress and negligee that I had bought
especially for our first time together. As I walked into the
bedroom, John patted the settee.

'Sit down next to me, sweetheart,' he said, 'you're just in
time. *Match of the Day* is starting.'

Later in bed, as I tentatively touched my husband's genitals,
I was shocked. I had expected his penis to be completely
covered in hair; instead it was smooth and warm and, erect,
an angry purple. Some time, during the following hours, I
told John what I had thought; he held me tightly and, as I
rested my head on his chest, he finally made me laugh. Our
shared sense of humour has carried us through worse
moments since.

Soon I relished the influence I had in being able to make
him grow strong and rigid; ready for our lovemaking, and,
away from the claustrophobic atmosphere of my mother and
father's house, I gradually learned to enjoy our shared
experience of sex. I trusted my husband and we were learning
about one another's bodies.

We continued to work in the Civil Service; life was good.
But after a few weeks I had a dilemma. These days it would

be called sexual harassment; in the nineteen seventies it was unacknowledged. The head of the section where I worked, a middle aged man called Peter Wood, took every opportunity to brush against me, touching my breasts as he reached past me to take out a file from the shelves where I was standing, squeezing behind me between two office cabinets to get to his desk, patting me on the backside, making sly jokes about sex. Unwilling to involve John, as we both needed the money we earned and I was afraid he would confront Mr Wood, I finally decided that the only solution would be to change departments.

But, one day, the problem solved itself. I was transferring some old files down to the archive room, a large musty area in the basement of the building. It was very cold, and the stone walls were whitewashed and flaking; there was ceiling to floor shelving around the room and down the central aisles. Unusually the door was not locked. As I flicked the light switch, there was no answering gloomy forty-wattage illumination. I remember turning to the trolley, picking up and carrying in the first box of buff coloured files, intending to put them on the floor of the first aisle and then report the broken light bulb. Suddenly I heard a bumping noise and as my eyes grew accustomed to the dimness I saw them. Rona, one of the typists, with her plump bottom on a shelf, had her thighs around Mr Wood who was breathlessly pumping away between her legs. His trousers were around his feet, his jacket, shirt and tie still immaculately fastened.

Then everything happened at once. As they both turned to look at me, shock on their faces, yet unable to stop moving, a huge pile of files fell from the shaking shelves that held Rona and scattered over them, I dropped my box of files and fled. As I ran down the corridor I heard the lift descending and I veered off towards the stairs. Two elderly typists emerged, chatting, from the lift and headed for the archive room. Breathless with laughter, I was back at my desk quite a while before Peter Wood came back into the office.

Instinctively I realised my problems were over and that night told my husband what had been happening. The unfair outcome of that episode was that Rona was sacked and Peter Wood got promotion and was transferred to another section. But for me, life in the office became pleasant again. Working in the same building meant sharing our lunch hours in the staff canteen and being home in the evenings at the same time.

However, by the time we had been married six months, I think we both realised our sex life was in a predicament. John often ejaculated almost as soon as intercourse took place and although I liked the closeness of sex, the tenderness it engendered, I knew instinctively that the briefness of our lovemaking upset him. Yet sex was not something we ever discussed. I think we both assumed that with practice, our lovemaking would improve. Our petting sessions when we were courting had never extended to any actions 'below the waist'. Going for counselling was never an option – my husband would have been mortified to speak about our sexual experiences to strangers and anyway we wouldn't have known whom to approach. So, even though I felt there was something lacking, I always reassured him that I was satisfied.

It was a lie. And as the months passed I became increasingly frustrated and angry. Our lovemaking never felt finished, complete, and of course it wasn't, but I didn't know why. We began to quarrel about trivialities. Neither of us wanted to confront the real problem. On my part, having been so humiliated by various events in my life, there was no way I was going to chance hurting my husband. Discussing it recently, he told me that he thought at the time there was nothing he could do about the problem.

Eventually we learned to prolong our lovemaking and I enjoyed the pleasant movement inside me; I accepted that. Until my first pregnancy and my discovery of masturbation.

Within three months of giving birth to our son, Sam, I

began to take the initiative. Finding the thrill of orgasm and the purchasing of a book I came across entitled *The Joy Of Sex,* resulted in John and I revelling in our own uninhibited sex. We had arrived!

But then, when Sam was four years old, I gave birth to my daughter, Shelly. I had gained a great deal of weight during the pregnancy and it was a difficult labour. After some weeks the heavy uncomfortable feeling in my pelvic region was diagnosed as a prolapsed womb and I was fitted with a ring that was supposed to keep all my insides 'in'. Not only did it fail to do its job, every time I coughed, laughed or sneezed the thing popped out and although our laughter was a bond, inside I felt humiliated, sexless, and John knew it. The body I had strived for, rejoiced in, in my late teens, that John loved, had gone forever. My breasts, previously large and firm, had been bound because I developed mastitis in the first week following the birth and I had been given tablets to stop the flow of milk (I was told I would be unable to feed my daughter, and for some reason I never questioned medical opinion!) and they were now floppy, as was the flesh on my stomach. I cringed whenever my husband touched me, conscious that he could be comparing my body with the one with which he had first experienced sex. Whenever he cuddled me, I rejected him. It was as though the last few fulfilling years had never existed. I returned to masturbation.

For the first year of Shelly's life, John and I had no sex life whatsoever. By this time John had had promotion at work and we had moved to Wales. As we had decided not to have more children, and I was still struggling with a prolapsed womb, I was advised to have a hysterectomy, and that a vaginal rather than an incision procedure would mean a quicker recovery. After the operation I developed bleeding in the peritoneum and lost a lot of blood, had to have an emergency operation and was very ill. During the following year I needed a bladder, a vaginal and then a bowel repair, a direct result of the first operation. Making love was not a priority for a long time. Whenever we attempted it, the pain was too great, so there followed a period of time when there was no intercourse. Gradually, though, our cuddling turned to the petting of our courtship days and then we gained sexual gratification through oral sex and masturbation of each other. Eventually we adapted to a gentler sexual routine.

Then I began to suffer from recurring clinical depression. John was supportive throughout my illness, but looking back I am aware that he became more my carer than my lover. It was during these years that on two separate occasions, I discovered a breast lump. The initial disbelief and fear turned to relief when each was pronounced benign. But, in turn, this resulted in an inward angry misery. More disfiguration! More reason to avoid being touched. Our sex life was at an all time low. But this time we talked for a long time about how we both felt and, after some weeks, reassured by my husband's gentle insistence, I accepted the body that was my life's inheritance.

Eventually, I learned to live with, if not always control, the depression, and when my daughter was thirteen I went back into the Civil Service. Most of my colleagues in the office were women and I relished the friendliness and also the sense of independence my work gave me. Over the next twelve months I became close to one woman in particular, Daphne, and we often went together to eat our lunch in the park; or, with a shared interest in the theatre, saw evening productions of the local amateur or visiting drama groups. Unhappily married to a man who worked abroad, she nevertheless had a cynical sense of humour that appealed to me. She was someone in whom I could confide and I told her something of my childhood. She was often lonely and visited us frequently. John liked her. One evening, after a night out, we shared a taxi home. We were laughing at some recollection of the play when suddenly she leant forward and pressed her lips to mine. For a moment I felt a quiver of excitement and returned the kiss. Her mouth was soft, enquiring and gentle;

her hand between my knees. I became aware that the driver was watching us in his mirror and, embarrassed, I turned my face away to look out of the side window. We didn't speak until the taxi drew up outside our house and I got out. I gave her my share of the taxi fare and she held on to my hand. As she started to get out of the car, I touched her shoulder and shook my head. 'We'll talk tomorrow.' I remember my voice sounded thin and stilted and as she leaned quickly back in the seat I knew then I had lost a friend.

When I went into work the following day there was tension between us and at lunchtime we automatically made for the park. It was one of the most difficult conversations I have ever had. I had to admit that gradually I had realised that Daphne was gay but still I allowed us to be close. I am ashamed that my curiosity let me test the feelings of someone I had great regard for and I am not proud of this incident. Whatever it was that I had felt when she touched me, I was unwilling to pursue it. I loved John and would never be unfaithful, but also my sense of survival was strong and I knew there was too much to lose, too much I had strived for, too much I had gained to make my adult life mine. I left the Civil Service and began working in the offices of the local authority.

My father died when I was in my mid-forties. Although it seems incredible now, I suddenly felt that I had no idea where he was. Instead of being two hundred miles away, living in the north of England, now he was in my head; he knew my every thought. The sense of freedom I gained when we moved to Wales was not just the experience of living in an area of open splendour whenever I looked out of the windows, it was also in the knowledge that I had escaped my past. My father's death changed that. Suddenly I didn't feel safe anymore. Every time John and I made love I saw my father's face instead, laughing as he held my arms above my head, his body heavy on mine, or 'that look' when I knew that whatever I said, however much I cried, it would make no difference, he would lie there, pretending to wrestle until he climaxed. As I write this, I am shaking. In the months after he died I was forced to confront the revelation of what he was doing to me as a child. It made me ill. I had a nervous breakdown.

For ten months I was on sick leave from work and struggled to survive everyday life. I coped within the confines of my family but attending counselling sessions and group therapy was tough. It probably was very useful but my only wish was to be at home with John and the children, my family. As time passed my apathy lessened, in contrast my sexual appetite increased, and making love confirmed a sense of our belonging to each other. Somehow all those scars and my changed figure became unimportant. I was at ease with myself and for a long time we regained the spontaneity and fulfilment of those earlier years

Then I found another lump and it felt different; the diagnosis that it was malignant numbed us. Our lovemaking took on a desperation – short, often frantic, shutting out everything except the effort of two becoming one, each giving strength to the other. There was no finesse, no slow dance of foreplay, just a frightened clinging together. Our days passed in automation; only at night in the dark were we ourselves, proving we were alive. But soon the clinical procedures overtook us. No longer lovers, we were just survivors through surgery, radiotherapy, treatment, medical opinions. Our lives were no longer ours. We existed only to exist, holding hands through diagnosis, prognosis. For a long time we lived without sex. It was unimportant to either of us.

Now, five years later, hopefully we are out of the tunnel. The drug Tamoxifen is a lifeline that takes us into the future. We are two people, boy and girl, man and woman who have matured together, a couple in love and companionship. We have realised that sex is not a perfect art. There are clumsy moments, disappointments, unfinished acts of love; but ultimately it is a statement of our love.

I no longer feel the need to masturbate.

As this work evolved I began to realise that I was going to have to show it to my husband. After all, my experience of sex isn't just mine; it belongs to both of us. We began this voyage together. Each of our acts of love has been different, through the lust of the moment, comfort in sadness and in grief, physical relief in times of stress, celebratory acts of triumph, affirmation of our love. It's been a journey that we have done together and I couldn't have had a better partner, friend and lover to walk alongside.

John tells me he has always known that I have masturbated at times; he understands why and if he'd known how ashamed I felt we could have talked about it long ago.

With his arms around me, I realise I haven't needed to carry any of the guilt all these years.

Discovery

KATHERINE DOWNHAM

One by one, each of us in the group was asked to share the myths we had grown up with about sex. A group of teachers and healthcare professionals training together to deliver an agreed LEA sex education syllabus, we were exploring ignorance, presumably to enable us to offer a sympathetic response to our students. I knew what I was going to say even as I listened to the shy and charming man who confessed to his fear of sex, based upon the belief that it was possible to become glued together. He had dreaded being carried into an A and E department on a stretcher joined to a woman in a compromising position, having become locked during the act of love.

I would confess that I grew up with, and even practically married with, the illusion that this 'act of love' only needed to be performed once. At the age of ten I knew *all* about sex. My mother had told me and, as I had a younger brother, I knew what a penis was. I did not know about erections or that sex was supposed to be pleasurable. But I was ignorant of my ignorance. Once inseminated upon one's wedding night, presumably a messy, floppy business, babies would follow in due course and life would proceed as planned. I knew that Eve had been cursed and imagined that this was the form it took. I did not yet possess the key as to how the babies were 'started' but that would doubtless be revealed to me later.

But it never was, because my mother died. So I grew up

with a very strange view of sex, knowing something of the mechanics but nothing of the emotions. I was told to save myself for that one special person but thought he would have to be pretty special to indulge in the apparently repugnant ritual of intercourse.

Having suffered a sort of arrested development as a result of my mother's death and a flirtation with a very comforting fundamentalist religious group, I married and was duly disappointed with sex. I was safely on the pill, anaesthetised by it and completely unimpressed. Many of the strategies used by disappointed women became an integral part of my life. It was easy to be exhausted. I was working full time; he was unemployed and at home with our baby. The baby woke early so that I could attend to her, and retired late, so that I could spend time with her. I had no notion of how much sleeping both of them did during the day, so that I could benefit from her company! The company of my adult daughter is preferable.

Exhausted, dispirited, rebellious, at the age of thirty-four, I met my liberator. I discovered sex, wild, irresponsible, guilty, orgasmic sex. My first orgasm at the age of thirty-four and it was simultaneous. What a revelation! I shared this pleasurable experience with a man who had no difficulty discussing sex and who was quite prepared to admit not only that he maintained his erection by silently repeating his Masonic oath but also that women often asked how he did it. There was no deceit. It was a brief, liberating experience.

Women often associate guilt with pleasure and I knew that I should feel guilty. Standing in front of the mirror, repeating the word 'adulteress' at my image and waiting for the lightning to strike, I only felt the urge to laugh wildly. I was enjoying myself. Later I suffered horrible discomfort as I sat awaiting the results of a pregnancy test, as I could only guess which of two men might be the father.

How did I find myself enjoying sex, when I had shied away from it for so long? Resentment played a large part.

Unusually, I had arranged to meet a friend in the village pub and was looking forward to the rare treat. My husband had tried to sabotage my plan by taking me to visit my sister in North Wales and returning late. I escaped, not too unhappy, as I was certain that my friend would be there and I would not be sitting alone.

I was propositioned and succumbed. After years of loyal, dowdy, dutiful domesticity and servitude, imagine being told that you are the most attractive woman on the (crowded) premises and then hearing a detailed testimony to his skill as a lover. Perhaps I should have insisted on being the most attractive woman in the county, but I lacked confidence. He had had a dalliance with my friend, of course, and probably half the women in the pub. I have no doubt that if my husband had not behaved so badly, I would not have had the courage to defy him and go out. When a woman is defiant she is capable of uncharacteristic behaviour. Though some might view my slip from the pedestal as sordid, it shaped the rest of my life.

Erotic and romantic film and writing, which I had believed owed more to the imagination than to realism, took on a new meaning and depth for me and when I encountered my irresistible present partner, we both fell in love. Sex and love in harmony are the very best that life can offer a human being. In C.P. Snow's novel, *The New Men*, Lewis Eliot observes a look pass between two people, the look of a couple who are completely happy in bed, and reflects upon his own unsatisfactory sex life. How long is it since I read that book and why is that small detail so well remembered? Because now I understand it and know why it tormented me all those years ago. It is a look I learned to recognise when I was forty and my life changed permanently. Old friends sometimes tell me that I sacrificed my career and independence in order to enjoy my second relationship. I say that it had more to do with my experience of sex.

40s

'. . . surely if the sisters were doing it for themselves it should be fun?'

The Feminist Guide to Spanking for Softies

SUZEE MOON

Would you be delighted to find such a guide? Pleased to indulge your secret fantasy? Require something a little less 'tame'? Or should anyone even mildly interested in such a topic be drummed out of the sisterhood? As this would be my sexual 'grail' you will appreciate my dilemma.

I am grateful to Maria Marcus, author of *A Taste for Pain: On Masochism and Female Sexuality*.[1] What was helpful was Ms Marcus's premise that masochistic sexual fantasies do not have to be part and parcel of a general masochism. On the dedication page of the book she quotes from *"Lilith's Manifesto"* in *Sisterhood is Powerful:*

> And Sister, if you can't turn on to a man who
> won't club you and drag you off by the hair,
> that's yours [hang up]. Keep your hang ups the
> hell out of this revolution.

---

1. I bought this rather 'textbook' tome in Hay on Wye. The male assistant slowly read the title, looked me in the eye and said, 'Shall I put it in a bag?' As the last book I bought was automatically bagged by him without comment I gave him the look and voice reserved for buying a nit comb, contraceptives or other such delightful purchases and said, 'Whatever – that would be fine,' and hoped I seemed more like a serious student of psychology than a sad pervert. I am also grateful to Barbara Wilson for her witty and serious look at feminism and sadomasochism in the lesbian 'community' in her highly entertaining but thought-provoking *The Dog Collar Murders*.

The thought of a sexual relationship with the modern equivalent of this Neanderthal stereotype fills me with horror. I am not naïve about real violence and have dedicated many years to both a women's refuge organisation and the rape crisis movement. My private sexuality, however, is fuelled by some very un-feminist fantasies. I tried 'regulating' my unorthodoxy, having read earnest articles on the subject in the days of *Spare Rib* along the lines of non-feminist fantasies being damaging and something the fantasisers should defeat/ outgrow. I tried, honestly I did. I'd think about my favourite topic and try to switch over to a more acceptable subject prior to orgasm. I guess the language itself is enough to tell you how unrewarding such attempts were.[2] I wanted to be a proper feminist, but surely if the sisters were doing it for themselves it should be fun? So I rebelled. The feminist thought police couldn't read my mind. Surely I couldn't scupper the revolution with my well-hidden, incorrect and saucy thoughts despite *Lilith's Manifesto*?

Those of us who wish for 'straightforward' sex in a heterosexual monogamous relationship are rarely questioned about the formation of our tastes but those who vary are more likely to be asked, 'So what made you – gay/swinging/into rubber/ an adult baby/a fetishist etc.' I love the term 'vanilla' to describe so-called 'ordinary' sex.[3] Like many who fantasise about variations I adore vanilla but think an occasional sundae is a treat. Sex has a great advantage over ice cream – as the brain is the biggest sex organ it's possible to think and talk sundae while 'doing' vanilla and you still get the fruit, nuts and sauce – try doing that with your basic ice-cream cone! I don't actually know what made me what I am, but here is a brief history and my attempts at amateur psychology.

---

2. I later learnt that these were methods devised to 'treat' deviancy such as homosexuality when it was illegal and thought morally degenerate. More recently it has been used with sex offenders. Perhaps I should be relieved I wasn't encouraged towards full aversion therapy and electric shock treatment!

3 .The term is used by those into sexual bondage, sadism, masochism, fetishes, domination, and/or submission.

I was born in the 50's and was brought up a Catholic. I was very shy and was bullied from a young age. I remember being so terrified of some children that I would do anything to avoid them. No thrills there. There were also children in my school who thought me beyond contempt and so ignored me. This meant I spent a lot of time daydreaming. As a Catholic I was well-versed in concepts of submission, 'offering up suffering',[4] sacrifice and tales of martyrs. Some clues, perhaps? I suspect, though, there are an awful lot of women brought up similarly who find my tastes peculiar. Although I did not comprehend the idea of sexual fantasy until well into my teens I had early fantasies of vague suffering at the hand of those who were somehow my inferior. My superiority lay in the nobility with which I bore the persecution – definitely a touch of the martyr! I also remember imagining scenes of spanking.

What was it about that word? It had a magic for me and the fascination of the unknown. As a child I didn't want to be spanked but found the subject thrilling. I know I hated pain. At home discipline was rarely physical. When it was, it was a hastily administered slap on the leg from my mother, which I hated and resented. My father never physically chastised me. At school the thought of the cane terrified me and I was thankful that it seemed the preserve of the boys (an early bit of sexism for which I was thankful). Boys usually got the cane on their hand but there was something exciting about the idea of bending over and receiving punishment 'Whacko' style. Most teachers commonly administered a slap on the leg or bottom but I never received one, as I was a 'good' girl. I remember only fear at the thought of rousing a teacher to slap me.

---

4. If Catholics 'suffer' something for no good reason (anything from a grazed knee to bereavement and serious illness – all very character building!) they are encouraged to offer up their suffering as a gift to Jesus who suffered for us to atone for our sins – This was *my* understanding of the things I was taught as a child.

The question that intrigues me (and I've never dared ask in case I 'gave myself away') is this: were the fifties and sixties full of spanking images or did I 'see' them because of a predisposition? Did the following 'make me' into somebody with these tendencies or did I simply notice them because of who or what I am? Nature/nurture – don't you just love it? The memories from my childhood include:

* Dennis the Menace and Beryl the Peril *always* getting spanked in the comics.
* The afore-mentioned "Whacko" films and similar '50's films on T.V. where the interesting, 'feisty' young woman is spanked by the man she loves and becomes submissive.
* Similar films where same type as above falls in love with the only man who 'dares' to spank her.
* Doris Day films where Doris is interesting and feisty then becomes a pushover in love. I'm not sure if she ever gets spanked but somehow it would fit the plot if she did.
* John Wayne spanking a young woman – no idea why.
* An episode of 'Bonanza' where an 'Indian squaw' is apparently badly behaved and is spanked (off-screen?) with a hairbrush. The hairbrush becomes a 'reminder' for her to 'behave'.
* A Superman comic in which Lois is apparently spanked by a Superman robot (for being too inquisitive?) and hides her embarrassing secret; then it is revealed that Superman himself meted out her chastisement but Lois doesn't know this.

I cannot guarantee the authenticity of my memories but the above are what I believe I remember and I've seen enough repeats and old films to confirm their truth in principal. So, sisters, did you notice too? Perhaps you were indifferent or indignant? Me? I tingled and still do.

The tingling continued. I would imagine scenarios where handsome men meted out punishments to naughty girls or women. While these secret fantasies were thrilling I didn't see them as sexual and I discovered my sexuality in a 'vanilla' context. Simply progressing to intercourse through the tortuous stages of 'courting' was as much sexuality as I could handle. And yet in a separate little world the spanking thoughts were there.

As I became more sexually aware I realised sexual fantasy was part of the sexual experience. Once a boyfriend described how he'd spanked a girl who had been 'harassing' him. I got the tingle. I got drunk. I asked him to spank me. He wouldn't. I tried to forget. After all I was drunk. I would not ask again. In retrospect he was a spiteful power abuser and bully.

At some point I decided there was more to this sex lark than what I got with my boyfriend and I knew women could enjoy themselves alone so I decided to experiment. No prizes for guessing my thoughts as I discovered the delights of solo masturbation. My youthful fantasies came flooding back with wonderful additions. I now knew about sex; being spanked by any man was thrilling but being spanked by a lover or a man who would become my lover was the ultimate turn-on.

As I got older I became aware that my tastes were not so unusual and I found better, more sophisticated lovers, yet still my secret fantasies stayed secret. Why? I couldn't risk being seen as weird or perverted and feared ridicule and rejection. And I was a feminist. I read the odd thing about fantasy and realised I probably was not the only one in this position but it wasn't a topic of conversation in my circles. And I knew about 'real' violence. I also knew about sadomasochism and the thought of torture was a turn-off:

> Pass the nipple clamps and torture guide?
> I don't think so!
> You want me to be your full-time slave?
> Fuck off!

You'd like to take down my knickers and smack my bottom?

Ooh, I'm not really sure. Will it hurt too much? What if I hate it? Um – Perhaps you'd like to tell me a little more about it? Can I get back to you on that one?

I'd also read the stuff about fantasy staying as fantasy – so was I asking for a damned good spanking or what? Again I wasn't sure.

I found myself in my thirties, unspanked and between relationships. I bought erotica and some racy fiction of a general nature. I bought my Nancy Fridays and found some fantasies that appealed and even some discussion on sado-masochistic fantasies being acceptable but I wasn't convinced. I still lacked the courage to buy the more specific spanking erotica I now knew to exist. I knew the 'pro' and 'con' arguments on pornography and if feminists couldn't agree on clear blue water between porn and erotica, who was I to decide? Did such stories and images degrade women? Would they encourage men to abuse women? Were the women in such pictures making true autonomous choices? You think this sounds like a lecture? Welcome to my confused little world! Despite the debating society in my head I made a decision.

I decided I'd like a sex life and I would get one in an honest, adult way. I would do it through the ads. I also figured as I was planning to meet potential sexual partners I could risk the fantasy. With trepidation I wrote to a man who listed 'spanking' as an interest. I explained my 'interest' and lack of experience and we arranged a rendezvous. My daring at this seemed as much excitement as I could handle. We met and talked and walked. I was relieved at his normality. We sat overlooking the Mumbles when he said, 'What's this about spanking, then?'

I reiterated my interest and fears and he promised to bring his canes next time. Knowing he knew gave my first vanilla sex with him a definite taste of the sundae. I was being fucked by someone who *knew*! And we were planning another meeting. And he was bringing *his canes*.

Could I cope with the reality? Yes. But I enjoyed the memory more than the event. I have an indelible recollection of driving to Aberystwyth to interview potential staff for a project being fully aware of my striped bottom and loving the incongruity of it. It was also very erotic. The relationship fizzled out as we had little in common and his previous relationship had encompassed paying his partner the insults and humiliation she enjoyed. More their thing than mine and so we faded.

I tried a few letter and phone exchanges with men who shared my fantasies but then decided to risk an advert of my own, emphasising interest rather than experience. I met somebody I liked and quickly came to love. He knew of my sundae tastes from the start. We were compatible and the relationship blossomed. We enjoy vanilla but we both know I enjoy sundaes as well.

Yet still I don't wish to be out, hence my admiration for Ms. Marcus. Knowing my lover knows is wonderful. But could I live with the knowledge that my friends know? Or my more earnest 'sisters'? Definitely not! What will it take to make me feel 'normal' about this one aspect of myself? I honestly don't know. Perhaps there is more debate than I realise, but my habit of secrecy and protection makes me reluctant to appear too interested. I could perhaps ask if anybody else heard that thing on *Woman's Hour* about sado-masochism. So, OK, Madonna sang about it but we all know the things *she'd* do for attention. Now if Jenni 'came out' that *would* have been a landmark. I can but hope.

And my unholy grail?

In ordinary erotica, I occasionally find stories and scenarios over which I have pleasure mulling. An unforeseen incident in a 'straight' novel makes my day, as does hearing the word 'spanking' unexpectedly. I have rewritten bits of *Gone With the Wind*, various romantic films, novels and fifties-style movies where a spanking would pep up the plot for me.

I recently braved the net. I was terrified of accidentally finding something nasty or upsetting. I was also nervous of someone, somewhere tracing me. (The thought police? Spies from the sisterhood? People who *knew me*? Let's not even *begin* to think about the neighbours! *Family*? What do *you* think?!) It was a confusing journey but I found some images and stories that I could add to my mental library and I didn't faint away. The heavier duty stuff appeared to be available to those who were willing to part with money and credit card details but that was fine for me. Seeing a knicker-clad bottom bent over with a male hand hovering was fun enough. There's only so much a girl can take when she knows vanilla is a good everyday treat.

And as for 'The Feminist Guide to Spanking for Softies'? I guess I'll have to write it myself!

REFERENCES

Marcus, M. *A Taste for Pain: On Masochism and Female Sexuality* Souvenir Press (E&A) Ltd., London 1981. ISBN 0 285 62497 0.

Wilson, W. *The Dog Collar Murders* Virago Press Limited London 1989. ISBN 1 85381 066 5

Friday, N. *My Secret Garden: Women's Sexual Fantasies* Quartet London 1975. ISBN 0 7043 3294 9.

Friday, N. *Men In Love: Their Secret Fantasies* Arrow Ltd., London 1980. ISBN 0 09 924970 7.

Friday, N. *Women On Top* Arrow Ltd., London 1992. ISBN 0 09 911161 6.

Woman's Hour Radio Four 17 April 2002.

Memoir of an Alien

ANON

You always remember your first kiss, with nausea, and then your first sexual experience. But what about the real first one, the failed one, the one I didn't remember for years?

Babysitting was a good hobby for a girl. You could earn money, have a night away from irritating siblings, choose what to watch on telly and even invite a friend. My best friend at that age had lots of babysitting jobs and I went with her on a few. We stayed the night sometimes, especially if it was a special night like New Year's Eve. This time was just that night and we were going to sleep over, in the lounge on a corner-unit settee, with our sleeping bags.

The kids were her department, and she soon got them into bed. The TV had on the usual variety shows of the 1970s followed by a Scottish special featuring Moira Anderson or Kenneth Mackellar. It didn't matter to us girls, we were going to sit up talking for most of the night anyway. We had some cheap fizzy wine and drank a toast to the New Year saying, 'Well, it's over now for another year,' in that desolate way that teenagers see their lives stretching out ahead of them. As if youth were a curse.

Soon after midnight, we switched off the lights and got undressed by the light of the moon streaming in through thin flowery curtains. It was a typical late sixties built bungalow with gaudy furnishings to match. Fumbling in the semi-dark with our backs to each other, we didn't dare sneak a look at each other's bodies because the thought of the other seeing ours was horrific. We talked in the dark, lying at right angles on the L-shaped leatherette sofa, so we could see each other's faces. We asked what our best feature was. She was tall and well-developed, but not so pretty. I was small and boyish in frame, and naive in matters of sexuality. She said her bust was her best feature, naturally. I said my feet. I sat nearer to her as we whispered our intimate secrets until we got on to the topic of kissing. Have you ever kissed a boy? We were both thirteen, of course we'd kissed boys. But I wasn't sure if I'd done it properly.

Yes.

Properly? How did you do it?

I couldn't explain.

Show me.

I moved nearer, naturally. There was no question of it being wrong, no need to be embarrassed; she was my best friend.

Go on, we can practise, she said.

So I leaned over and kissed her. She was kissing me too and it felt . . . right. It was soft and natural, there was no passion, but I didn't feel repulsed, breathless or invaded. It was just right for a first kiss. It went on for a few minutes before we broke off unnaturally, unlike kissing a boy when his eagerness and yours means you can barely stop unless you are breathless. I could see her white breast almost uncovered in the half-light. It looked full and smooth. More than I had seen before, more than I possessed myself. I don't remember touching it, cupping it. But I remember that it was heavy, it looked heavy and marble-like in the moonlight.

I enjoyed the kiss. Then I went back to my sofa, went to sleep and we never spoke of it again.

It wasn't long after that that I went away with my family to a holiday camp. There were five of us kids, so, being the eldest, I was put in a chalet on my own. It was a sort of beach hut, two steps to the door, with its own toilet cubicle, wash basin and a single bed under the window. Some of the girls I met up with came to have a smoke there sometimes but there were plenty of other places to hide from your parents. These girls seemed to be more attractive than me. They were street-wise and wore big shoes and long flared trousers. They would look at my clothes and ask, 'Do people dress like that where you live?' The boys wore high-waisted trousers and could dance better than me. The boy I liked on first sighting paired up with one of my fashionable friends. So I looked elsewhere.

There was one boy who was OK but wouldn't have won a prize for his looks. His acne saw to that. Trying to catch his eye was difficult, he never seemed to be in the places that teenagers hung out. He was 18 and went to the bar with his dad. One day, near the pool, I took his jeans and ran off with them, putting them on over my bikini. I thought he'd see me as a lovely thing of beauty in a pair of jeans far too big for me. It didn't really work, just made his mum and dad laugh.

One night returning home to my chalet I met him going to his. It was now or never so I took the plunge. He happened to be in a chalet like mine in the same row. Oh, that's where you're staying, I said. I'll be round later. He didn't believe me, I could tell by his expression. But I wasn't going to pass up the chance, for what, I wasn't sure. So, well after midnight, I put my coat on over my nightie and went round and knocked on his door. He answered the door in jeans and no shirt, incredulously letting me in. Innocently I went in and we sat on the bed, under the window just like mine trying to make conversation. After we started kissing we were lying on the bed, in a rather uncomfortable position, him on top of me. My legs were firmly together, probably because I didn't know what else to do. His body was muscular but spotty, so not as smooth as I'd have liked, but no worse than anyone else I'd kissed. I still had my jacket on and as that began to come off revealing a little girl's nightie, I remember thinking, this is going to be it. I didn't even take my sandals off, those unfashionable things that didn't compare with the other girls' platforms, but this, was this more fashionable than them? His hand reached my breasts, underdeveloped but still there. He was squeezing them uncomfortably, but then I didn't know what was supposed to be happening anyway. And then it happened. I thought – this is it, if this is it, then, this is it. It's really happening. It just happened. No fireworks, no feelings of love, no pain or discomfort, just a feeling of it being slightly wrong but not knowing where to stop, or how to stop it. It was soon over, without any sense of build-up or climax. He was no great shakes, there was no foreplay, whatever that was, it may have been his first time. I didn't think about that. I hadn't even thought about opening my legs. I assumed it could happen without that. They'd lain there motionless for the few minutes it took. Afterwards I left. I needed to sleep, so we kissed and left it as if we would pick up again tomorrow. Strangely, I felt as if it would perhaps fade like a dream.

The next day he was with another girl, one of my friends, the best friend of the girl who had gone off with the first boy I'd spotted. So I didn't tell the other girls. There was a great feeling of having joined some exclusive club. If only he hadn't spoiled it by going off with her. My mum remarked on how sweet they looked together. I just nodded. But I decided not to let it go altogether and later tackled him about it. I said that he knew it was wrong and I could report it. I was well under age. It would be your word against mine, he said.

At the age of sixteen I had long fancied a boy whose brother did a paper round for my mum. He had left school, was now eighteen and because he was so much older and had never spoken to me at the bus stop when he was at school, I thought he couldn't possibly be interested in me. His mum was a friendly woman and asked me did I want to bring the paper to her house in case I bump into him? It was surreal because I don't think I had even mentioned him to anyone. His brother, who was my age and I think secretly carried a torch for me himself, fixed us up together and we met on the street corner.

He had lovely long dark wavy hair and a beautiful face with dark brown eyes, and just a slight imperfection in the shape of his face, but so pretty that you didn't notice it. He was slim, wore tight-fitting Adidas T-shirts, the ones that became associated with Man United in the late 70s, and tight-fitting flared jeans. The fashion was for Brutus or Falmers. I wore Falmers with the plaited strips on the pockets or the zips across the back pockets and they flared out from the hip. I also had a new red T-shirt, tight-fitting with a keyhole neck and a stand-up collar. We walked quite a long way to a pub that was quiet and we had a few drinks and talked. The Stylistics were on the Jukebox and the Floaters with *Float On*. He told me how he had always thought I was pretty but had been too shy to ask me out. When we left he put his arm around me all the way home which was nice. We kissed around the side of the house. It was the best kiss I'd had, well, for a long time anyway. It was that feeling of instant love, love at first kiss, that makes every girl tingle and soon I was having sex with him on his mum's sofa when his parents were out. I was totally in love with him and it would last forever as far as I was concerned.

One evening as we lay on the sofa, his top off, mine adrift, I was caressing his manhood very carefully and gently as always. Such a smooth thing didn't need much friction, it would have spoilt it, I thought. He was getting warm and moist and I thought it was part of the excitement that he was oozing thick warm liquid. It carried on with no sign of him getting any more excited, no build-up. Playfully I rubbed my sticky hand on his chest and opening my eyes to look up, my expression turned from laughing to horror.

It was blood. I had smeared red blood all over his chest which had been bleeding from his penis as I had helpfully pumped it. At that moment he suddenly felt the pain he should have felt from the outset and dashed upstairs to clean himself up before it went all over his mum's covers or carpet. It seemed like ages, as I washed my hands in the kitchen sink, before he called down that it was torn. I had torn his foreskin. I honestly don't remember being rough, but the guilt was terrible. More than that, I was thinking, no sex now for days, even weeks. He had to put a plaster over the end and take it off to have a wee. As this involved pain every time it wasn't long before his mates at work noticed. Then foolishly he happened to wince in front of his mum when he caught himself on the furniture. She asked him what was wrong and he said he'd done something at work. You want to claim for that she said. I think being in an embarrassing place helped him avoid pursuing it any further.

It wasn't long before normal service was resumed, but I got bored quickly. I got a Saturday job in a supermarket and started seeing someone there just to try out someone else for a while. I didn't like him much and had the chance to get back with my previous boyfriend, but it wasn't the same. I think that knowing I could be bored and tempted by others made me realise it couldn't be for life, anyway.

Chase

GWERFYL DELAHAYE

In a loft, dedicated to my father's addiction to clutter (and littered with the remnants of schemes to make him rich, stronger and more clever), I found pictures of young, naked boys, as well as of naked men and women. I lost respect for him.

In a car in Llandinam, packed with my cousins, one of them explained in graphic detail that girls bleed every month because their fathers prick their vaginas with a pin.

In 1969, my father bought a lime-green Dansette record player, along with records by Jim Reeves and The Supremes. I listened to 'Baby Love' by the latter group, and felt very profoundly (for the first time in my life) the urge to have a baby, and it made me feel exceptionally squirmy. Is sex merely the puppetry of procreation? I flirted outrageously with my brothers whilst playing 'Baby Love' as loudly as possible. Fed-up with my writhing dances, and jealous of the world I was beginning to journey towards, they retaliated by telling me that Dad might be ready to insert the pin. I ran outside to the cowshed (knowing intuitively that my cousin had it all wrong) and stayed long enough for them to think I'd discussed this difficult issue with my father. But thinking about the consequences of the subsequent story, the lack of suffering and intrigue (I had seen cows and bulls at it), made me determined to stick with the original and go for an extended horror version. I made them glad they were not female and enjoyed the stolen glances of wonder at the bravery of women and their fate.

This new power needed testing. The next object of my desires became the sixteen-year-old farm hand, Austin. Games of chase, tickling and eye contact, while parents were not too far away, ensued. Then the greatest, scariest and naughtiest moment of all was devised by my ten-year-old mind. I told Austin to look up at my bedroom window as he left for home one night. As he turned to look, there I was in all my naked glory, posturing provocatively, trying it out. Then my mother walked across the farm-yard and I threw myself backwards onto the bed, blushing and laughing with shame and delight. Things moved on quickly after that. We kissed in the haystack, Austin reassuring me that my breasts were growing and checking his statements with gentle fondlings; the games of chase improved, particularly the catching part. Gradually Austin metamorphosed into an extra brother and our intimacies fell by the wayside. I think he started going out with a girl his own age. There was nothing more I could imagine I wanted from him.

Living on a farm afforded a female child many mothering opportunities: diseased kittens stolen from a neighbouring farm because they were threatened with drowning, hen chicks, calves to suck your fingers while they drank milk from buckets, runt piglets and lambs to save by warming them in the slow oven of the Rayburn. Baby rats and mice, purloined from their mothers by my brother and his dog, were kept in my bedroom in my underwear drawer, fed with a doll's bottle, and inevitably died. To add to this catalogue of infant animals, there was the baby rabbit that was doing so well, until the cat got it: only half a skin lying across the Scaletrix track under the bed was left to remind me of its former glossy little self. So much powdered milk, made up into so many bottles, so many rubber teats thrust into so many mouths. Having recently discovered my own little teat between my legs and not really knowing what to do with it, I nevertheless found that putting milk powder on it, and letting puppies lick it off, was exquisitely pleasurable, but a bit dangerous if anyone caught you at it. My parents would have been ashamed of me, and I did not want to lose the higher moral ground gained against my father through my secret delvings into his papers. My brothers would have gained even higher moral ground, and used it mercilessly to their advantage. This was a secret to be kept (one whose pleasures were not re-awakened until my mid-twenties, when an affair with a well-travelled artist introduced me finally to the exquisite tracings of the human tongue on the clitoris and the deep chaotic orgasms that are its quarry).

As I quickly took on a woman's form, I found a further form of power, the envy of other less-developed females. My friend Molly (whose kittens I had rescued from certain instant death, only for them to endure a slow drawn-out one with me) asked for advice, and was informed that feeling them lots worked. This advice was given in good faith; I did feel my breasts a great deal, being exceptionally proud of them. They were my primary erogenous zone. I never learnt to masturbate (until the awakenings experienced in my mid-twenties led to desperate explorations) but the dreams that ensued from my fondlings sometimes led to orgasm, often preceded by images of primitive, aggressive and beautiful black men, dancing. At this stage of my twelve-year-old life, I had never met, or come into contact with a black person. The Supremes were the nearest point of reference, but my dreams conjured up male versions of the dynamic trio. We had no television, and rarely travelled further than the nearest market town of Newtown.

The next passion I explored was kissing and like many before and after me, the pillow became the mouth I practised on. The object of my desires, Twm, my second brother's best friend, filled my dreams, in which I conjured frothy weddings and babies and squirmed, sighed and lusted after kisses and cuddles. Twm and I experimented in the hayloft during games which involved Twm's sister Eirian pursuing my eldest brother, and various other children, my youngest brother amongst them, pursuing us to get a look at the kissing. I prided myself on my technique, not too slobbery, delicately moist lips, fitting closely and gently on to Twm's; our breath was always sweet.

Secondary school afforded a whole new heady range of conquests, but somehow the experience I had previously gained was forgotten and I began again. It was a strange, aggressive start, that began with attacks on older boys, so that they would chase me. I was at this stage a wild, dishevelled little heathen, who took delight in squirting water (with used plastic syringes once filled with a preparation for cows who suffered from mastitis) down various boys' necks and whacking them in the region of their genitalia as I whizzed past in the hope of initiating dangerous games of pursuit. My eldest brother despaired of me, told me to brush my hair, and tidy myself up. So my cartwheels and chasing games came to an end once more and youth club, 'Yr Aelwyd', and the second era of the older man as sex object began.

With my teenage years began an addiction to cigarettes (No. 6's), smoked in gateways, by fields, with posses of village children and one older girl who ruled the roost and handed round polo-mints so that we wouldn't be found out. I befriended another older girl, Gwenda, who drove her dad's car. Gwenda and I spoke Welsh to each other and she confessed her passion for a farmer in a neighbouring village. Huw Dolau was tall, dark and a gentleman of twenty-three, who wrote poetry and had a good singing voice: I respected him. Gwenda and I would attend 'Aelwyd' events (quizzes, table-tennis matches and whist drives) for the sole purpose of getting Gwenda hooked up with Huw. I acted as the clownish, charming go-between. Meanwhile, I espied, with my little eye, a twenty-one-year-old man, with mischievous brown eyes and a definite interest in this precocious thirteen year old who cruised around with Huw Dolau's girl. We shared Gwenda's car, with herself and Huw in the front and me and Wyn in the back. Blissful explorations of mouths, torsos and his penis ensued, with lots of long meaningful gazes into each others' eyes, which seemed to mist over in more passionate moments. I discouraged his hands from travelling beyond my knicker elastic as I had very little confidence in that part of my body at this stage in my life, whereas I knew he'd be impressed with my breasts, because I was. I loved to hold him close to me; the glorious tension of unrequited sex was a drug I played with, to get him hard, sweaty and panting out his desire for me (I had spied on my older brothers and their friends enough to know what the penis likes to have done to it). He never forced the issue of intercourse so I suppose he liked it too.

Our relationship was based on car sex, afternoon assignations in country lanes, moments snatched in Gwenda's car after an 'Aelwyd ' event, usually with another couple for company, who were up to the same things as us. From conversations with my friends I guessed that several of them had tried fingering, which I found slightly disgusting, but also fascinated me. I was finger raped at a Twmpath Dawns, the latter being a regular feature of rural life in the 60's and 70's. Wyn's brother, an unstable, deeply possessive man, had recently split up with his girlfriend, and we had both drunk too much cider. I hadn't seen Wyn for months and so assumed he'd lost interest. Elfed picked me up and led me to some dark corner in a nearby barn, the cider made me careless, and Elfed was bent on some kind of revenge on womankind. He ignored my breasts and pushed his hand roughly down past the boundaries of my knicker elastic. I told him not to several times, but he was very strong and I was very drunk. The shock of his finger thrust into my vagina was confusing, both sexualising and horrible at the same time. We hadn't really kissed or exchanged any intimacies and despite being drunk I felt angry, afraid and stupid. I found some energy and ran back to the dance. Everyone was leaving. I remember being sick and nothing else about the rest of that evening. I felt dirty and ashamed the next day and we never spoke again.

At fourteen, I began my first job in Lipton's, living in a front room which belonged to someone I had never met before, who also worked there. I remember little about the work, but I think it was a lonely experience. It was a summer of familiarising myself with pub culture and sad academics and salesmen who drank too much and tried to impress precocious young girls. This all happened at The Angel, which all of the drinks-, drugs- and sex-motivated populace of Aberystwyth passed through at one time or another, in the early seventies. People would sit on the pavement outside drinking cheap pints of scrumpy and those in the know would move onto Pernod when they progressed unsteadily inside. The sad thirty-year-olds would be manipulated by my smiles, flattery and pert young body, and buy me all I could drink. This game went wrong a few times, but I escaped relatively unhurt and wised up considerably. The first time a very tidy salesman became attached to me, I laughed inwardly, and smirked triumphantly at my friends, as he bought me drink after drink. Losing my sense of reality, and becoming quite drunk, I thought I would treat him to a little unrequited sex around the back of The Angel. We started kissing, but he was cold and sweating and his neat jacket, shirt and tie seemed so out of place, I giggled. I could not take what we were doing seriously, and I gratified my desperate urge to pee by squatting down in front of him. This action disgusted the tidy salesman, who proceeded to shout abuse. He shook me roughly by the arm and I thought he was going to hit me. I returned the abuse, and asked him what he was doing with a fourteen year old anyway, which was a bit below the belt; I had played a very convincing eighteen year old all evening with him. He was furious and shocked. I left, running all the way home. Lipton's had a pleasurable mundanity about it the next day.

The second incident was fuelled by my constant desire to impress and shock myself and others with my conquests of older men. I despised them for their compliance. I think I really wanted a strong-minded older man to give me fatherly advice and rein me in. But there were and are so few fathers.

Paul was in his mid-thirties, bright blue eyes, too short, usually dressed in a shabby suit (I think he had a job) and he drank a lot. One night, in the usual haunt, the flattery and flirting routine began: the drinks were bought and Paul became more attractive as the alcohol took hold. We ended up on the beach, that gritty, grey Aberystwyth beach, and I suddenly found myself with a man who knew a lot more than all the others. Paul knew how to turn a girl of fourteen on. I was surprised and wrong-footed; he appreciated my torso and moved beyond the knicker elastic. This was not in accordance with my life-plan; I was determined to remain a virgin until I met someone better than this. A flash of reality (this man is thirty-six, pissed and shabby), several refusals to go further, my observation that he wasn't really hard and his messy ejaculation on my stomach, freed me from any attachment to Paul for ever.

The next night, as the bar of The Angel began to fill up, some girl friends came over to say that Paul was spreading it around that he had shagged me. My adolescent outrage knew no bounds. I stormed up to him. 'You have no right to say that you shagged me, Paul! You did not! How dare you say such a lie! You're a fucking prat!'

I did not wait for any retort and strode out feeling morally superior and gratified by my outburst. Ultimately I felt defeated and restless, so I retreated hurt with a Chemistry student, who was nineteen, overweight and rather ordinary. He never excited me enough for me to get angry or surprised, but he offset my excesses with punctuality and reliability.

From the age of ten onwards, I had been aware of my parents' misery as a couple and often implored them to get divorced and get over each other. Now, I did not make things easy for them. One night I did not come home. Because I was only fifteen, I had had to work on my mother to let me go to a concert in Shrewsbury and come back on the late train. A friend had procured two tickets for Thin Lizzy, and offered me one for free. Angrily and resentfully, my mother caved in. I became intoxicated with the music and the various drinks, and Marie and I danced like fiends right in front the group, exchanging flirtatious glances with them and the occasional yell of appreciation. I had never been so close to famous people before, and the lead singer, Phil Lynott, was the first coloured person I had observed in real life. After Thin Lizzy's set, another group came on and I suddenly decided to try and get off with one of them. Marie already seemed to have nailed her quarry and we were both on a power trip, exultant and full of expectation. But when invited to a party, I felt I wanted to go home. I had a train to catch, I was satisfied with the conquest, and offstage they reminded me of Paul, of his shabbiness and limitations. Marie had no qualms about missing the train, but I insisted they would have to take us back to our village, reminding them it was quite a drive. It turned out that the party was halfway towards home and I reluctantly agreed to go.

The drive to the party was high-spirited and we all drank beer and smoked. I began to fret about getting them to drive us home. Marie was on another planet, laughing and kissing her newfound trophy. We arrived at what seemed a deserted farmhouse. But there were about eight of us, so it seemed lived-in after the initial rituals of getting fires going and opening more bottles. There was a double bed with half a curtain slung around it for privacy. Marie and I ended up side by side with our respective trophies, mine no longer really wanted. My plan was to give him a little bit of the old 'unre-quited' and then hope for a lift back home. As I ran my hands over his torso, and rubbed his cock, I realised he was quite drugged or drunk. Marie's partner on the other hand was slipping his cock into her and going hell for leather. This was the first time I had witnessed live sex, and I was strangely shocked. Marie seemed very passive, and not surprisingly she was asleep as soon as he got off her. I panicked (I'll never get home at this rate, everyone here is out of it, hardly able to speak, let alone drive). I brought a reluctant and doped penis to a mild shudder of ejaculation, and began demanding a lift home. I had no money and there was no phone in the house. At 5 a.m. I gave up, slept fitfully, and woke as an angry, desperate colossus of determination. The van lurched its way to the village, the urban group making wisecracks at the simple country scenes they observed, with their hung-over and doped eyes. We stopped well out of sight of the village. I was too ashamed to be seen at such an early hour of the morning attached to such a motley crew. White-faced, relieved that I'd got away with it, once again, I prepared to meet the wrath of my mother (my father was often away) and instead was met with her tears. We shared cigarettes and a rare emotional exchange. She was desperately worried that something had happened to me. I assured her it hadn't.

The following summer, I persuaded my mother to let me work in a hotel in Aberystwyth. One of my friends was distantly related to the owners. We lived in a run-down house at the back of the hotel along with a motley collection of students, unemployed people and a family who should really have been in some kind of sheltered housing scheme. They had exceptionally low intelligence and were vulnerable to the exploitation of the hotel owners, who operated some scam with the Social Security people. They worked long hours and the owners somehow convinced them that their board and lodgings equalled their wages. The young girl was used for sexual relief by both a student, Guto, and a young unemployed man. Her bedsheet would be patterned with a scattering of wet patches on some afternoons, and the smell made me gag. We accused Guto of not caring; as a student we thought he was out of order leading her on. He shrugged, said she didn't complain, and grinned inanely. The mother, a bedraggled, untidy woman with a few bad teeth left in her mouth, lived with a bewildered and scrawny nineteen year-old. They talked about their sex life a lot, which mostly happened in the attic of the house we lived in. One day she showed her bedroom to my friend and me. Aside from a bright pink cover, it was like a putrefying version of Tracy Emin's installation, 'My Bed'. Very early on I drank too much sherry at a party, and moaned about the loss of my former boyfriend, Wyn. I fell over lots and pissed myself in bed and it took a week for me to recover. My mother visited me and called me a slut; there was something refreshingly direct in her statement and I did not defend myself.

Richard was tall and blond with intensely blue eyes, a student of geography with a penchant for acid. I stayed with him overnight. I adored the sensation of cuddling up to a naked man: it was a tender and exquisite exploration and the rule of unrequited sex was adhered to. I was punished the next night for this. Calling round at the house after work, I walked into a party in full swing. Richard was snogging some girl amorously; he glanced at me with a momentary flash of both sheepishness and defiance, and carried on. I felt like kicking him and crying at the same time. Instead I had a drink and attempted the brave face technique, chatting to friends whilst thinking how lovely my first night spent with him had been. I couldn't quite believe that what I was watching was true. After they left for Richard's bedroom, I too made a quick exit, mortified at his callousness. The next week was spent conquering another man who belonged to the group of people who lived in Richard's house. I wasn't interested in him, but I wanted to make Richard jealous. Davie was good-looking but his life was totally predictable. (I still see him about – I was right.) But he served his purpose and Richard and I were soon back together. Physical explorations of each others' bodies continued to fascinate me and although he asked from time to time for penetrative sex, it was never a real problem. He enjoyed the way I played with his body. I had become an expert at diverting men from penetrative sex. Richard proposed to me a few months before my sixteenth birthday, but I told him it was an unfair question to ask someone so young. He then became more interested in acid and one afternoon I saw him in the distance with his face bruised and scratched and his hair looking as if it was pulled out on one side. I lost interest.

A year later, I met a very tall man and fell in love for the first time and lost my virginity. Afterwards, this man did not believe that I had been a virgin, which I felt was a bit of a shame as I had spent so many years protecting myself, ready for the real thing to happen and be the beginning of something new and fine. His first love and wife had left him and so he did not trust me. I tried to leave him before his mistrust and revengefulness engulfed me, but, just like my mother and father, I did not have the courage.

In 1978 in Prague I had an affair with a Bulgarian actor. He was impotent. In 1980 I had an affair with a married man, and played the old game of unrequited sex. His wife phoned one day, and scared the shit out of me. In 1982 I had an affair with an artist. I played the old game with him and he gave me wonderful oral sex, which is why I kept seeing him. I did not like him, he reminded me of a hungry dog. Later someone said he had been in love with me for many years. Now a sort of sad guilt rules my life. Everything is 'unrequited'.

Contrasts

ANON

'I blame it on the pills,' is my husband's frequent refrain. OK, the side-effect sheet did suggest that a rare occurrence could be loss of sex drive, but when I stopped being able to orgasm with the frequency I'd previously enjoyed, it didn't stop me still wanting to make love and being satisfied. However, my man was On A Mission: the wife must reach the big 'O' each time we had sex by hook, crook or forefinger. Now no one has been able to achieve the finger method except me so I rapidly went off sex altogether, as did my husband.

Then I met the man who became my lover. We'd been working in a group one evening a week for a couple of months before I really noticed him and then I gave myself a stern talking to after he smiled at me and my insides did things that forty-something women should put down to a dodgy curry. During the last week four of us were working intensively together during the daytime and he made his move. Wherever my sex drive had been hiding, he found it. His kisses were warm and dry, hard and as urgent as the monster erection I could feel on my back as he spun me around and fondled my breasts and held me to him. I ran my hands down his lower back, buttocks and legs and arched my back so that I could kiss him along his jaw line. I was in orbit; we fitted together like pieces of a jigsaw. He was just that bit taller than me so that everything felt in the right place. As we couldn't find anywhere private where we could go and see how things developed, the last three days with the group were torture. We had to act normally when all I wanted to do was rip his clothes off. A wink from him and I was wet with longing. At home I was trying to act normally. Not! Sex had become a ritual to be got through as soon as possible, but my husband had reverted to his mission – until I told him it was impossible. I just couldn't tell him why. He kissed wetly, and bit the inside of my mouth; I realised where the expression 'having one's face chewed off' must have come from. As for cunnilingus, I would squirm in agony rather than ecstasy and be grateful that he couldn't see my face! As I get most satisfaction being 'on top' that is where he liked me to be, because he got off seeing me enjoy myself. But it was getting difficult when I was trying not to think about someone else.

About a month later I met up with my lover. He came around to do some work on the house and obviously chose a day when my husband would be absent. We warily moved around each other while he sorted his stuff out and I showed him what needed doing, then suddenly I was in his arms and it was like I'd never been away. We collapsed onto the sofa and explored each other but he couldn't wait, and I wanted him pretty badly too. He warned me, but even so, I had never seen anyone so big, and it was only the fact that I had had two children that I wasn't scared stiff (I left that bit to him . . .) He was so gentle and strong and came so fucking quickly – the occasion had overcome him too. The rest of the time was spent just holding me (in between working, called coffee breaks!) and caressing me. Of course, he had to return the next day to finish off what he had started, in both senses, and we had half an hour of delicious screwing in several positions before we succumbed. His normal expression is quite serious, but he has a killer smile that he doesn't let loose very often. It's enough to make me come on my own.

My husband has magnets in his hands that automatically zoom to my tits when he gives me a hug. Or my groin. That is not what I mean by 'Gissa hug'. Also he has to suck my neck which makes my toes curl, and not with passion. I've recently lost weight and toned myself up and he fancies this new me. He is soft, though not overweight. My lover has only ever known me like this; he is a physical man, hard, muscled, strong but gentle when he holds me, whereas my husband uses his strength without realising, holding my upper arms to pull me to him so that when I resist I end up bruised; squeezing me instead of caressing. I suppose I must have liked and accepted it once, never having known anything different. Now I have been spoilt by something better physically. I know I am not his only lover by any means, but we don't talk about that. He laid his cards on the table – take me as I am when you can but don't bring love into it. Show me a woman who wouldn't try and change his mind.

We have X-rated phone calls – thank goodness for mobiles – and it's nice to be told that you are wanted and have the evidence graphically described to you; 'my lunchbox has just levitated by 8"' was the best!

'So put it on the dashboard,' was my reply.

My husband loves me and I know that I turn him on. Sadly, he hasn't turned me on for some time, even before I met my lover, so for the moment I am playing with fire and lust and while I enjoy the fun times, it's gonna end with a bang in more ways than one.

Melted Down to Stars

SIÂN MICHAELS

> *"If love wants you: if you've been melted*
> *down to stars, you will love*
> *with lungs and gills, with warm blood*
> *and cold ..."*
>
> from *Last Night's Moon* by Anne Michaels

One of my dearest friends is eighty-four, and still shocked every time someone offers her a seat on the bus or tries to help her cross the road. She's tiny, knock-her-over-with-a-feather tiny, wrinkled and shrunk; like the hand of time is already preparing her to be preserved, pickled, a specimen of age. Shocked? She's outraged! So she should be, anyone with more than a second to look at her face – soft, mischievous, framed by a fluff of hair that must have once shone gold, lit by eyes so blue they hurt to gaze at too long – that this is no old lady. This is a girl of eighteen: fresh, lovely, vibrant. How dare they treat her like an old lady?

I know how she feels. The mirror lies. This face – forty-one indeed, with the audacity to look back at me as though it were my mother – is not mine! This body! I'm tiny, like my friend Eve; time didn't need to shrink me – I've never made it to five feet. So slender that my slim fourteen-year-old daughter can't fit into the green silk dress I wore for my graduation ball. Neither can I. That is to say, neither can that person in the mirror; the one with stretch marks across a stomach that looks like elephant hide, drooping breasts and a waist that, as my Gran used to say, is 'a waste of time'. That can't be me. I'm a girl of eighteen: fresh, lovely, vibrant. How dare those towering teenagers call me mum?

Me and Eve: eighty-four, forty-one. It makes no difference; we're still the same inside, girls of eighteen, and, when the lights go out at night, I don't even have to pretend, don't have to scurry deep inside myself to find her. Age has done its worst in the daylight, but not in the dark. It has not penetrated my night-time mind or my pussy. Only Craig has. One man, over and over again.

He comes to me every night now as he did when I was a girl, raw with apprehension as we lay in the sand dunes looking up at the night sky, shivering even though it was warm.

'Everything comes from the stars,' he told me. 'It's a pretty violent beginning, but it's how things get together.' He grinned, brown eyes mocking and hungry. He rolled me onto my back, pinned me down with his body, his hand reaching under my thin cotton skirt.

'Cataclysmic explosions, supernova, then matter flung out into the universe.' He laughed, buried his face in my neck, kissed it, hard, watched me melt, his hand reaching inside my pants.

He's large, Craig, six foot two, broad, with hands like great shovels roughened by work. They are potter's hands now. In the daytime I watch him coaxing the day into shape. He's patient, so patient, but resolute; the largeness of him bent in wrapt concentration over the emerging shape, slowly getting what he wants out of it. His grey hair is just a mask. In the dark, in my mind's eye, it will be fair again: a shock of unkempt curls.

When I was eighteen, chronologically eighteen, I understood sex, understood it with my cunt, deeply, instinctively. It was fire and water and air. I had never felt so vulnerable, never felt so powerful. The good girl, the clever girl, the girl who would go to university and get out of this place, joyfully tearing off her clothes to let Craig in. His friend had a flat; my friend would cover for me. God, it was good!

Craig had a way of coming up to me from behind, holding me so tightly I could barely breathe, so certain, so confident, his large hands loosing their grip after just a moment, knowing I would stay still, that I didn't have to be told. I would breathe in quickly, shocked every time at the exquisite loss of control. Acquiescence assured, he would lay me down, and lie behind me, one arm caressing my naked back, the other under my head reaching up to fondle a nipple. Another quick intake of breath, and I would begin to writhe, but only to feel the sharp sting of a warning slap burning my buttock.

'Shh, lie still, be good . . .' His voice would be soft with humour, but urgent. 'You know you want it.' The fingers on my nipple would twist, a tiny motion, almost pain, electric, quelling me into indecent compliance. 'That's better.' Craig's laughter was like perfumed oil, soothing and subtle. 'Now . . .' He'd roll me onto my front, slipping a hand under the damp mound of pussy. Fingers would lick their way inside me, teasing my clitoris, enlarging the moist space inside me, until I came in a crescendo of rapture, my breath ceasing completely before returning again in thrilling gasps: Craig would laugh, his cock hard and hot against my thigh, teasing, tender, in control. 'Little slut,' he'd whisper, 'you know you can't resist. My little plaything is what you are.' He'd flip me over and push into me, relief and ecstasy breaking across his large, smiling mouth. He was never gentle, but he was tender, his hands running over my nipples, his mouth searching out mine in engulfing kisses, or biting into my shoulder, marking me. I would come again, crying out at the exquisite delight of so much exposure, so much gratification. Then Craig would come, drenched in sweat and we would collapse together, like puppies in a heap; indulged and replete. We were grateful, not bootlickingly grateful, but in awe, that there was another human being in the world to whom we could safely expose ourselves. Because we were exposed, stripped down far beyond naked-ness, far beyond fucking, to the bare bones of our desire.

Then, at eighteen, I was naive and ripe and melted easily. By the time I was twenty-two, I knew a bit about the world. I'd been to university. I'd watched people who fucked: soulless, joyless stuff that couldn't touch what I did with Craig, or savage shagging that was all about display and conquest, nothing personal. I didn't want what they had and I didn't want what the prim Christian Union students had either – all that self-denial, all that longing sublimated into extempore prayers that made me shiver with embarrass-ment on their behalves. None of that could melt me, but, still, I was seduced: ensnared by unselfconscious, confident youths who could quote a poem or dive into the dizzying cut and thrust of debate about politics, God, art or gender. I was fired up with the terrible righteousness of the young. I could see it all now – Craig was my oppressor, the bastard, telling me I wanted it, making me melt into submission, having me spend the whole weekend playing the part of his 'pleasure slave'. Well, no more!

By the time I was thirty we had three children. Gravity and childbirth had taken their toll. Politically correct sex was such a bore, but it was all my re-formed mind could allow and, anyway, I may not be one of those evangelical die-hards who tell strangers in public places that they love Jesus, but by then I had joined the church. A woman deacon and mother of three could hardly dress only in silk and gauze scarves and play the slave, agreeing to obey her husband's every sexual whim. Well, could she? A feminist theologian who knows all the tricks of patriarchy all the way back to Adam can hardly purr when her husband spanks her till her backside stings and she promises to be good. Well, can she?

I wasn't eighteen anymore and I knew it. Craig kept his

distance, made do with occasional offerings in the sanctioned mode. When I looked into the mirror, I saw the disapproving face and sunken, all-martyr eyes of my mother looking back at me. I saw the unrecognisable body of some fat, frumpy woman regarding me with scorn.

Then I met Eve. The world, taken in by her alias, thought that she was seventy-eight, but Frank knew better and I knew better too. I watched her. She had a body that was visibly getting shorter year by year, a tiny slow-growing malignant mole over one eye, a heart condition that made her dizzy and slow moving and excruciating arthritis that fed her lifetime insomnia with pain. On one visit she showed me the letters that Frank had sent her when he was forced to work away to make ends meet.

> *'Darling Eve,*
> *How I miss you . . .'*

> *'My dearest Eve,*
> *I think of you all the time . . .'*

The mundanities of life on building sites, the bed and breakfast places, the anecdotes about workmates were spattered with words of longing and sensual affection

'That was when we were young,' Eve smiled. 'Just about the age of you and Craig.'

Young? I was thirty-five. If Craig worked away there would be nothing much to miss. We shared the cooking, shared the chores, shared the inactive bed. Eve's blue eyes shone with adoration as Frank entered the little living room. His long body picked its way through scattered postcards and letters, carefully balancing a tray of drinks and biscuits, without Eve missing a movement.

'There you go, Eve.' He passed the china teacup with reverence, their fingers lingering on each other's paper-thin skin as she took the cup from him. 'Biscuit, Sian?'

For four years I watched Eve. She was my parishioner and I was full of compassion, fetching shopping, taking her and Frank on hospital appointments, fretting over her as her body got smaller and the pains left dark rings round her lovely eyes. She was not ashamed to show adoration and gratitude to a man. I was fascinated, drawn in, more seduced by a quiet old woman than I had been by those ebullient students.

I remembered Craig touching me the way Frank touched Eve – tiny, familiar movements that only intimates could understand. What we had was shabby and tired by comparison, the occasional connection that had all the passion of cheap, damp fireworks: a little promise, not much delivery, no hint of melting stars. Somewhere between political correctness and the sleepless nights of parenthood, somewhere between religious calling and making ends meet, we had lost what we had.

Five months I spent in bed, so ill that some days the exertion of getting to the bathroom was too much. At Christmas the children bought us a great bag of luminous plastic stars and stuck them onto our bedroom ceiling. At night they glowed in the dark, thin green lights, soft, but cold. We didn't melt. Occasionally we fumbled towards each other, awkward, restrained and cautious. Craig didn't laugh or say much; they were undemonstrative encounters, functional conjugations. For eight months more I was sick. I lived a day at a time, a few good days, plenty of bad. Craig took on all the cooking, all the cleaning, got up early to work in his downstairs office, never mentioned sex.

I went away on retreat at the end of thirteen months of illness. I caught the train at five in the morning and finally arrived at the Abbey fourteen hours later, cold, wet and aching with fatigue. I tramped up to the Abbey from the ferry, too late for supper; I was thirty-nine and felt old, older than Eve. I was there to convalesce, to rethink my life, to soak up the beauty and spiritual balm of the place and

face my future. What would I do? I might work again, but
not in the church. I'd blazed a trail, the first among women
priests, always dynamic, always challenging. I'd campaigned
relentlessly, fought the good fight, but illness had stripped
away the masks: superwoman, working seventy hour weeks
and still making time for her children; the activist, banging
on the doors of patriarchy till they let me in; the advocate,
shouting for the poor, especially the women and children, a
string of groups and forums and charities left behind me.

'You brought so much love to this place,' Eve had said
every time she visited.

I had been so loved. Changing the world for God was
better than sex. They'd loved me until I was ill. They with-
drew then, let down, angry, their own needs so raw that my
vulnerability was an unforgivable offence. How could I
have needs? How could I be weak? How could I hurt?

Eve had called every week. 'You brought so much love to
this place,' she persisted, but I had to wonder: where had all
that passion come from? Sex sublimated into the love of
God? While Craig waited on the sidelines, grateful for the
crumbs that fell from my altar?

At the Abbey, I missed Craig. I had known that I would
miss him, his reliability, his patience, the hundred little acts
of generosity that made up every day with him, the presence
of his solid warmth by my side at night. I missed all of that,
yes, but more than that, I missed sex. I missed the sex that
we had had for those few years at the beginning. The sex
that had been an enormous shock, like a cold ocean wave
hitting my face, taking my breath away, and leaving me
panting, shivering and disoriented.

It was cool in the chapel, the sound of the sea a distant
lullaby. Pilgrims came in quietly, full of reverence, one by
one or in small, hushed knots of friends until the place was
full. The words were Celtic-crafted, poetic, lulling. The
music was lyrical, as soothing as the candlelight reflected
off the stones, as comforting as the soft red wine brimming

in the earthenware chalices beside the new-baked loaves. The service swirled around me, familiar cadences suddenly empty of meaning, once lucid hymns suddenly a cacophony of babble.

'Though we pass through tribulation, all will be well . . .' Will it? All?

'Faith may seem like a mystery, it seems like folly, it seems absurd . . .'

I wanted to scream back to the preacher, 'Seems? There is no seeming about it! Sacrifice? Service? What about life? What about sex?' But I said nothing.

I was eager to return to Craig, as eager as he was surprised. 'What brought this on?' he asked for months. They were hard months. We had to leave the vicarage. We had to uproot the children. We had to make ends meet on so much less. 'What brought this on?' Nothing we had to solve could shake me out of this new resolution to become eighteen again. I had known what it was to melt like stars. I had watched Eve through all those years. I had survived illness and had my epiphany, alone, in a sand dune, miles from home, outside a little Abbey, watching the stars. I could be sick or overweight. I could have greying hair or ageing skin. I could have stretch marks and sagging breasts. I would still be eighteen. 'What brought this on?' I only smiled and climbed into bed.

Retreat from Eden

ALICE WINTER

My experience of sex began in a rose garden attached to the local common, at the age of eleven. He was gorgeous, black and eminently grown-up. I was with a friend, and he'd followed us all the way over from the seats by the sundial where he'd earlier been occupied chatting up two other young (though to my eyes older and infinitely more sophisticated) girls.

He appeared, seemingly out of the blue, on our bench under the arbour. I felt complimented: he was sitting next to me and all his attention, everything he asked, was directed towards me. We exchanged ages. He was twenty-one. He offered me a cigarette. I refused. Then a crisp from the bag he was holding. I took one. Then he kissed me. A full on crispy-tongued, alcohol-soaked kiss, his left hand pummelling feverishly at my chest. I was more turned on than I ever had been before, or would be to this day. And that's when the panic set in.

I rose suddenly urging my friend to join me, and we began a quick retreat down through the garden along the edge of the common to the bus stop. He was following us. We dived into a phone box and feigned a call until our bus came, then made a dash for it. We'd lost him. Only I hadn't.

The palpitations followed me home. I tried to clear them by getting up my little portable 'dansette' record player in the middle of the living-room floor, and playing my favourite single of the time over and over and over. I danced like fury, but it made no odds. There was no avoiding the fear. The guilt. The desire. Even now, some forty years since, it takes no more than a couple of bars to bring the whole thing tumbling back.

From that time onwards, sex became a way of life. But not fun. Just a cycle that all too quickly became too powerful to break: a premature adulthood that progressed into a pernicious round of pain, drugs and consequent depression. It's only now, in early middle age, that I am finally beginning to come to terms with the idea of sex as a source of harmless, guilt-free pleasure. This has proved to be one of the saddest and most damaging journeys of my life, both mentally and physically.

And, yes, I do hold him responsible.

Frustration, Over-ripe Bananas and Other Myths – A Confused Adolescence in 70's South Wales

SUE JAMES

For a girl born in 1955 I knew a surprising amount about sex – everything. And this was as a pupil in a Catholic junior school living in Sarn. When my sister was born in 1960, I knew she'd been inside my mum's tummy. I knew all about babies in tummies and where they came out, although I admit I was a *little* hazy of quite how they did it. I had, after all, pored over the pictures of tadpole-like and monstrously-headed unborn babies. Why, I even knew they were called *foetuses*. Not for me the birds and the bees – straight to the real thing. The *Virtue's Household Physician* was a real boon to my early education. Luckily I hadn't stumbled on the horrifying section graphically illustrating the terrible consequences of venereal diseases, including the dire warnings against the sin of Onan (look it up for yourself – I had to!) known as self-pollution. If I'd found this information earlier my mother would have had a more challenging time answering my questions.

I think it was when I was about ten or eleven that my ever-logical mind found a few puzzles to mull over. I was used to this. I was always coming up with theories to make sense of the confusing world. It occurred to me that something had to start the baby off. That was easy. It had to be God; after all he was responsible for everything else, wasn't he? Then there was this thing about unmarried mothers talked about in hushed tones. I knew The Blessed Virgin Mary was sort of one but that was because of God – but then so were all babies, weren't they?

OK. God 'started' babies and he'd make it start by . . . what? You were supposed to be married, but what about the unmarried mothers who were not the BVM? So it was obviously something you did when you were married and not when you were single, except by accident. Why, it was obvious! It was simple proximity that did it. I thought briefly about brothers and sisters but of course God was clever enough to make them immune. You'd think he could have done something about single people who got pregnant accidentally but perhaps it was one of those things I couldn't *quite* get to the bottom of . . .

So come eleven and secondary school I knew all about it. I recall a conversation between Ella and myself in form one. We both admitted we knew all about babies and Ella said that children *as young as us sometimes had babies*. At the time I was sometimes convinced that on hearing something for the first time *I'd already known it.* 'Oh, yes,' I agreed, 'wasn't it awful,' and we both tried to imagine the unimaginable. It got a little wilder as we tried to outdo each other regarding the youngest mothers. I think one of us 'remembered' hearing about a four-year old . . .

I later tried to fit this into the puzzle. Pregnant children, too, were the result of getting too close to a man or boy. Luckily I had no reason to worry. The boys despised me and I didn't have any brothers. But there were a few girls who spent an awful lot of time with the boys who were still in junior school. I'm not sure how I refined my theory but at some point I realised that beds were significant. That made sense. God would decide to make you pregnant at his will if you were married and shared a bed. Unmarried mothers were those foolish girls who lay on a bed with a boy . . .

In form two I hated boys. I had good reason to do so – they hated me! My friend Clare, however, was extremely fond of boys and often snogged them. I got a bit worried after one such session had taken place on a bed and Clare told me the boy had joked about her getting pregnant. I joined her knowing laughter but worried that she could get pregnant; especially when I realised the grown-ups had noticed her liking for the boys and muttered darkly.

The next step in my sex education disturbed me greatly. We were on holiday in Porthcawl and I was in the loos with my mother and wanting to throw something away. She pointed out that there was no bin and I disagreed. I pointed to the sanitary bin and was told it was a special bin she would tell me about at another time. I was filled with a mixture of curiosity and an inexplicable foreboding.

That evening I found myself alone with my mother and knew I just *had* to know. Somehow I already knew I wouldn't like it but as ever curiosity won out. We went back to babies. Yes, *of course* I knew all that but what on earth had babies to do with bins? I listened in horror as I learnt that babies needed *blood* and women produced blood every month 'in case' there was a baby! Worse was to come! It wasn't only married women and mothers but *all* women. *Then* I learnt the worst! It could happen to *me* at *any time now* and would happen *every month*. How unfair was *that?* The bins were where you put these disgusting bloody pads you had to wear when you were away. At home they were burnt. The following day I went to the loo, saw a spot of blood, ran to another cubicle and threw up.

Somehow I came to terms with the terrible reality that was known as 'periods' and started to notice the pulled faces at 'the time of the month', packages wrapped up in news-paper, smug girls allowed to miss P.E., especially swimming, and mysterious burnings when Dad was out of the house. It took me a few years to realise my father and other men actually *knew* about periods. My new knowledge also put me off buying family blocks of ice cream – similarly wrapped in newspaper by the thoughtful shopkeeper. I couldn't *possibly* explain my aversion to fetching the Sunday treat I so adored. My demand for a shopping bag was granted but I still had the fear that someone could come into the shop *after* the wrapping and *before* I got the ice cream into my bag.

At about thirteen I knew about men having seed and women having eggs. Thanks to confusing jokes and rude comments this eventually fell into place. Somehow out of the ether I acquired the knowledge that men put their penises into women's vaginas and made babies. Yeuch!

Meanwhile the whole world was courting and getting off with each other. Boys and girls made crude remarks and actually showed an interest in this sort of thing. I didn't know who were more stupid – the horrible boys or the girls stupid enough to fancy the horrible boys. Now if boys were like David Essex or Leonard Whiting I could understand it. I was too clever to think my heroes could possibly be interested in a mere schoolgirl and I knew that those convinced they were made for David or an Osmond were just plain stupid.

Clare didn't moon over pop idols – she snogged real boys and talked about feeling sexy and was fascinated with the idea of 'going all the way'. I was horrified but didn't show it. Going to the Catholic school was enough to brand me a snob, without looking down my nose at girls who managed to get off with real boys.

When Clare wasn't getting off with boys while I covered for her we were members of The Red Cross. Very worthy! By now Clare had outgrown the charms of triangular bandages and improvising splints from handy umbrellas or walking sticks but she stuck it out. It was, after all, the gateway to socials with the Bridgend group and a whole new load of boys! There were no boys in the Bryncethyn class.

I, too, made an interesting discovery in Bridgend. Boys who didn't *know* I was an object of contempt treated me like a real girl! I could be normal. OK, they were no Leonard or

David but they *talked* to me. My role as Clare's cover continued and the only way she could see the latest love of her life was if I was there as well. It was fine when we were at an actual event at Bridgend but accompanying her to the town and whiling away two hours on my own was not something I was prepared to do more than once. So Clare had her grand idea. Apparently her current swain had a friend who fancied me. To Clare's disappointment I wasn't enthusiastic but I did agree to go to the next 'Red Cross disco' with him.

It was OK and I agreed to get some fresh air with him – I was fourteen and had never had been kissed. I knew I had to get this right. It started off as merely interesting – this kissing lark – but I was a bit startled when he tried to get his tongue in my mouth. I knew enough to know this was 'French kissing' but I was not impressed. He didn't seem bothered so we reverted to a primmer form of mouth-to-mouth. So this was it. Nothing to write home about.

When I agreed to go to the cinema and make up a four-some I actually allowed a little more intimacy on the mouth-to-mouth front. I was, however, convinced that the contact of his body against my breast was accidental and he hadn't realised what he was doing.

Several boys later and more obvious attempts to touch me forced me to revise this opinion. I was also increasingly aware of boys' states of apparently permanent randiness when around girls. I got used to fighting off hands and protecting my virtue. I discovered other girls besides Clare talked of randiness and 'giving top and/or bottom' – references to touching permitted. I was horrified – especially when the talk moved to the subject of inside or outside your clothing and having your nipples sucked – but then I was a prude from the Catholic school.

Despite my outward Puritanism, sex fascinated me. I could read about it for hours – and sometimes I did. I would have passed any theory test on the subject by the time I was sixteen. I'd read the lot – or so I thought. Not a million miles away from the kid in juniors who'd also known everything. In the seventies an awful lot was written on the subject. I remember being very amused as a teenage virgin reading an article in the *Mirror Magazine* debating whether 'good girls' should be told about sex. As a good girl reading it for myself I appreciated the irony.

What made me uncomfortable, however, was the realisation that I wasn't as 'above it all' as I'd like to think. I would never discuss *giving top or bottom* but I found I liked attention paid to my breasts and it made kissing more exciting – including French kissing. The disadvantage was having to keep up my guard to ensure no further liberties were taken. I kidded myself my boobs were not getting deliberate attention but the thought of actually putting a name to further activities in the confessional box probably played a part in my discretion.

At sixteen I found myself once again making up a foursome so a friend could spend time with the boy of her choice. My mood was very much one of 'doing a favour' and when I found myself alone with John I wasn't averse to a kiss and cuddle while the others disappeared upstairs in Patrick's otherwise empty house. John was not the best catch but he was alright and I think I must have decided to get the most out of the encounter.

I let my imagination roam and enjoyed the kissing without thinking about the kisser. When my breasts were touched, I carried on enjoying the sensations in my own little world and managed not to 'notice' as he unbuttoned my dress. I felt the expected shiver as he brushed over my bra and held my breath, as his fingers were the first to explore inside my 'armoury'. I somehow managed to ignore the reality of the boy as I gave myself up to the pleasure of the feel of his mouth taking over the earlier attention he'd paid my breasts. It was wonderful. Then he attempted to get his hand up my dress. I leapt up, pulled my dress together and blustered.

And then it happened.

'Fucking prick tease!'

And I knew he was right. In my arrogance I'd let him go 'too far' and now he was out of control and of course it was my fault. I'd let him do unspeakable things and now I was paying for it. I was lucky he didn't 'make me' 'go further' – after all it was my fault! Hence the reasoning of a good South Wales Catholic girl of the seventies!

Luckily my secret stayed safe and he merely walked off in disgust. I didn't blame him. I *was* a prick tease. I just had to ensure no one else discovered it. And so began the next stage of my 'education'. How to go out with boys, keep them interested, not be a prick tease, not be a slag and not be a snob . . .

As a teenager I'd discovered the youth club attached to a neighbouring school where the boys didn't automatically treat me as a pariah. I just had to be careful not to come over as a Catholic snob. I refused to have a 'boyfriend' as I didn't want to have to make difficult decisions about sex. I did, however, 'get off' with lads and agree to further dates where the action was limited. I have weary memories of fighting off the wandering hands along most of the route between youth club and home. I took walks into the forestry, along the railway and the playing fields, attempting a balance of pleasure, normality and chastity. It was a difficult act but I maintained my chastity.

Eventually a boy who was handsome, self-confident and could make me laugh battered through my defences. I explained I refused to 'have a boyfriend' but was willing to go out with him so he increased our dates until he was seeing me every evening I was free and meeting me from my part-time job and other activities. I knew I was weakening and having proved I wasn't 'easy' allowed him the liberties I'd avoided since being labelled a prick tease. He told me he was 'frustrated', as had his predecessors, but I was unwilling to go further. Then he told me he loved me.

This was a dilemma. Although I was scared of going all the way, I too felt excitement at our limited activity. And I loved him. The pressure mounted and several things made me reconsider. I knew nice girls didn't and it was a sin. I also knew we loved each other and that he had got so desperate he nearly did it with my best friend. I not only forgave them, I took the blame for his unhappy state! I truly believed unrelieved frustration was harmful for boys. I remembered vague jokes and comments about overripe bananas and explosions, which I'd only half understood. I also truly believed in the romance of saving myself for marriage (sexual liberation took a while to reach some corners of South Wales). And now that we had declared our love he was my first boyfriend, at the grand old age of seventeen.

So the pressure mounted. We were secretly engaged. He loved me but couldn't bear to be near me because of the 'frustration'. It would make him moody and he couldn't bear to kiss me because of the 'frustration'. It seemed he was permanently aroused in my company – how could I not be both flattered and guilt-ridden? I just wish I'd known that this was the normal state for teenage boys and not my personal responsibility!

For the first time I agreed to touch a boy 'down there' and was completely astounded at my first sighting of a penis. It appeared to have a mind of its own and was a strange mixture of the intimidating and the absurd. I found the attention it required intriguing but within my powers to grant. It was all a bit odd but it meant that my secret fiancé no longer had to avoid contact with me because of his 'frustration.' This was, Dear Reader, a mere step on the road to my full initiation.

Now I'd touched him, he wanted to touch me. I'd *never* touched myself there for pleasure in all my seventeen years. It was only a year since I'd finally got the courage to insert a tampon. And everyone knew nice girls didn't do that sort of thing. I knew that the limited attention I'd already received was exciting so I realised going further would probably be thrilling and the idea of genital contact no longer struck me as weird and absurd. I was worn down by his desire rather than my own. It did feel good but it was a while before he was able to improve his technique and relax me enough to make it really good.

But I took to mutual masturbation and oral sex and joined the ranks of the knowing, sexually experienced technical virgins. It was exciting but it was still about him. I still had to fight off his attempts to go all the way. He was no longer frustrated but wanted the 'ultimate' because he loved me . . . I genuinely wanted to hang on to my virginity because it was more romantic and full sex was definitely a sin. I was knowing enough to know the sexual activities I already practised were beyond the pale but, like many others, my actual lack of intercourse was very important to me. I knew the Catholic Church, mothers and the problem pages of most magazines would smugly declare that 'if he loved/respected you he'd wait' but it all rang hollow. Because 'the adults' didn't talk about the things I actually did for my fiancé I was able to live with the unspoken knowledge of its wickedness and damp down the anxiety of not being as 'good' as I would have liked to be.

And of course his desire to go all the way continued. I find this extremely difficult to acknowledge and admit today because it seems so absurd. I usually say the following as though it is a joke. It wasn't. I prayed. I didn't want to go to hell. I loved him. I would have liked to believe he loved me and would do so if we were not having sexual activity but this was my reality. This was the man I was going to marry and despite my best efforts he was still in agony because of my refusal of the ultimate. I also knew that if I considered it a sin and did it anyway there was no salvation because forgiveness was only possible through perfect contrition.

My solution was not really a satisfactory one but as I had to balance impossible choices I came up with a fudged solution to make sex outside marriage *not* a sin. I convinced myself that as we intended marrying it was OK and only circumstances stopped us being married already. It was a fudge and I knew it but I could live with it.

In theory we hadn't *definitely* agreed to do it but we decided I should go on the pill 'just in case' – an ordeal in itself. The Bridgend Family Planning Clinic was in a building that was once, so I later discovered, the Work House. Now it was doing its bit to stop the birth of foundlings rather than give them dubious succour. In the seventies, despite the 'sexual revolution', all visitors were called 'Mrs' – this was years before men were welcome at such places. I dreaded being found out.

Bridgend Family Planning Clinic was probably prepared for a lot of things but they hadn't considered the attendance of a seventeen-year-old virgin who wasn't planning for her honeymoon. They assumed I was experienced and puzzled at my inability to cope with the insertion of a speculum. I moved higher and higher up the couch in my misery but unable to articulate my dilemma. Finally the doctor solved my 'problem'.

'When did you last have intercourse Mrs James?'

'Never!' in a relieved, embarrassed squeak.

They decided not to persist and I left clutching my three packs of the pill.

Of course, he agreed we didn't *have* to do it, but we were both aware of the dawning of day 14 when I was safe. And of course we drove to 'our spot' on the common car park in Porthcawl. And of course we did it. And continued to do it.

And once we made our decision and I knew I was going to continue to have sex I was determined that I would make the most of it. I enjoyed the thrill of it and my power over him and found his endless desire for me exciting. We were seventeen and did it *everywhere*. What could be more thrilling than mitching school and *fucking* in the sand dunes? I have memories of wandering around the dunes with my school blouse open having just done it and knowing we were about to do it again. In this first sexual relationship, the very excitement that I was not only having sex but was also, in my own eyes, very sexually sophisticated, seemed enough. My reading, however, made me aware that there was more to it. The odd orgasm I'd had before intercourse also made me aware of possibilities but somehow most of the time I measured my 'sexiness' in terms of *his* excitement and my daring. My moment of silent rebellion finally came following his excitement at an article by Germaine Greer on 'women on top'. I was quickly fucked and then thought, "Is that *it*?" I squashed the thought and went for a pee. After all I loved him, didn't I?

At college the relationship continued and I measured it in quantity rather than quality, proud of the fact we sometimes did it *five times*! I was now au fait with the idea of female masturbation and occasionally performed for his pleasure but was secretly proud of the fact that I never did so on my own. All my reading, however, was filtering through and discontent eventually surfaced. My sex life was exciting but wouldn't it be fun to see if I could give myself an orgasm? For some reason this thought came to me as I queued to take out books from the College library and my long-squashed, but vague youthful fantasies about arousing a man when he was tied up bubbled to the surface. As a child, and more recently, I had thought taking off my clothes for the helplessly bound Superman or David Essex thrilling, but now I knew a lot more tricks. There and then, in the library queue, I decided I was going back to my room to play with myself. And I did. And it was fabulous. And it was secret.

When he finished with me he broke my heart but luckily it mended and I went on to be a contented serial monogamist with some very lovely men and only the odd encounter with a bastard. I discovered the things I liked and began measuring quality rather than quantity, although I treasure memories of those first few heady months of a relationship when the sex seems endless and there appears to be a need to stand downwind of others in case the waft of satisfaction literally assails their nostrils. I adore having sex in a loving relationship with someone who knows my body. I also found my first explorations of one-night-stands as a thirty-something quite an experience . . . but that's another story!

30s

'A strange wet-fur smell wafted up from under the duvet. By then Ravel's Bolero was long over . . .'

Two Beds, Four Heads

ANON

From somewhere in the club Miranda had managed to get hold of a partner for the night, though she must have been under stress because he was well below her usual standard. He was called Hannibal, which didn't suit him. He was black as usual, but as a rule her one-night stands were older, cooler, just physically bigger than her. Hannibal, however, was clearly an innocent and, it transpired, a virgin too. In retrospect, he and I would have been better matched – but I had my own appointment to keep.

And he was at the house already. I managed to avoid his eyes as we set about task one: moving the double beds together. Miranda's mother was away as usual. I can't remember when we decided to move the two beds together, but by the time we arrived home there was no budging the idea. Hannibal and Sam did most of the work. It was one of those terrible pink divan bases and we had to shove it on its side, rucking up the powder blue shag-pile carpet all the way into Miranda's bedroom. Then she had a sluicing session in the bathroom while I went to prepare a snack. When I arrived back, she was in the red kimono with Sam's arm round her and Hannibal was sitting on the other bed on his own looking bemused. All I remember now about Hannibal is his grin and his overwhelming desire to please. He didn't say very much.

Miranda put a record on her battered deck, did a couple of languid swirls in which her gown flashed open, and snaked her way towards the bed. Leaning on her elbow she started to massage my shoulders, 'Hey, poor baby's tense. Just relax, listen to the music.'

Ravel's *Bolero* was winding itself up slowly, weaving round the houses; I got up. 'I need the loo.'

'I'll keep you company,' said Sam from the bed.

'No thanks! I'll see you in a bit.'

I put the lid down and sat on the toilet in peace, looking at the bathroom for what seemed like the first time. Everything was white; even the carpet had been white, but now there were half prints of people's feet graffitied onto it and it was black with mildew in a line by the bath.

The shelves, windowsill and sides of the bath were jam packed with women's products: all sorts of delicious miniature freebies and exfoliating things; a scrubber on a beech wood stick (with short hairs clinging to it); two jars of bath salts: one lemon, one pink; a glass bowl filled with glistening bubble bath balls; a brand new real sponge in its hessian bag; a spaghetti jar full with pastel-coloured cotton wool balls. Miranda's cap box was there too, open like some great oyster shell. I'd seen her cap – it was the size of a saucer. I was just tidying up the things on the side of the bath, putting them so the labels faced outwards and wiping off the dust with a damp flannel, when someone shook the door.

'Are ye ready?'

'Err . . . yes, fine, I'll be out in a minute.'

Flushing the toilet for appearance's sake, I went to wash my hands. There was still some soap left round the Imperial Leather label. It must have been bought by Terry, the mother's lover, or even bought in honour of him, because it was totally incongruous in that place.

'Are you coming Sue, or what?'

'I'm coming. Course I'm coming.'

'Well, come on then!'

'I'm coming!'

I looked at my face for just a moment before I slid back the bolt. I was beautiful in this light, even I could see that. No, I didn't have spots; I had big eyes, slanty eyes all dark and a long neck like a woman in a picture. It was now or never.

The bolt was small and mean, set up just to pinch your fingers but Miranda was waiting for me, pushed the hair back behind my ears.

'I've just arranged that!'

'Sorry.'

'What's'e doing, anyway?' I asked.

'What've *you* being doing you mean. You've been ages!'

'Tidying up. I've been thinking.'

'Too late now! Come on they'll think you've fallen down the loo.'

'I wish I had've.'

'Oh just get on with it. Get it over and done with, will you!'

She was right. It was getting beyond a joke! I'd been sixteen now for ages and *still* a virgin.

We made our entrance. Sam was sitting (well, lounging) like a Roman emperor on the bed. Since I'd been out he'd taken off his leather jacket and jeans and was wearing a red, sleeveless T-shirt and boxer shorts ready for business. They were a new invention and I guess they were better than Y-fronts, especially on someone his shape. He was obviously smitten; the job I'd done earlier in the week with the five scarves had been a real success. Remembering the grand finale, I pulled my elasticated skirt up under the loose top; he smiled, looking rat-faced, looking like some randy villain in a Catherine Cookson novel. There was something nineteenth century about him, something of the Bill Sykes. He'd always been seedy, even at thirteen.

As far as I could tell Hannibal was naked under the other duvet, quite handsome actually but the gormless expression spoilt it. He had lovely shiny shoulders and giggled as the elastic of my skirt made a snapping sound over my breasts.

The light went off – Miranda's doing.

For a moment Sam looked like the negative print of himself a moment earlier. Miranda's form passed me and landed with a flump on her mattress and there was nothing for it but to move through the yellow light from the street towards her mother's bed. Sam had the covers pulled back for me. The warmth of the bed, its softness, his arms all round me, was for a moment a huge relief. It was dark under our duvet; him ruffling my hair, hissing my name. I kept my legs curled up away from the fungus at the bottom of the bed. Already there was a bouncing noise coming from the other one and loud cooing noises – it sounded as if Miranda was in there on her own.

'My God, she's coming already!'

'First of many, no doubt,' Sam laughed. For a moment I'd forgotten she'd had him first.

It was quite cosy talking like this; after all he knew her too – was still going out with her in a way, though at his request temporarily on loan to me just long enough to end the virginity. He was kissing me, lapdog kisses, which seemed to be missing the lips and causing a sort of friction burn around my mouth. He was lying on me too, an elbow boring into my left breast. I didn't want to put him off his stride by saying anything so I just moaned encouragingly and ran the palm of my left hand up his inner bicep (or where it should be) and wriggled my hips a bit but it didn't seem to work – he ground down on me even harder, gnashing his front teeth together. I could see his eyes were closed. He was supposed to be good at this; he was two years older, after all.

I continued rubbing my palms up and down his body for a bit and had succeeded in shifting his elbow off my breast when he lurched off me, filling the bed with cold air. A strange, wet-fur smell wafted up from under the duvet. By then Ravel's *Bolero* was long over and Sam's shadow looked grotesque in the mustard-gas light: the shape of a mediaeval jester's hat strapped to his groin.

As he picked through the records Miranda surfaced from under her quilt and then Hannibal. He looked thoroughly dishevelled, lolling in the bed with a dazed expression.

Miranda had him lying across her chest, face up, her hair all over him and one arm over his torso like a tabard. His head lay on her left shoulder and was gleaming with sweat. I could see it, even in this dim light. They were the dead spit of the little mermaid and the drowned prince except for the fact that the 'mermaid' was rather too robust.

Sam hadn't seemed to find a record and his silhouette had changed significantly when Miranda piped up, 'Just stick the Ravel on again; it's seductive anyway.'

'But it's been on 60 times already!'

'So what! Have you come to listen to records or what?'

The *Bolero* started up again and he came back to bed clutching a cushion to his groin. His body felt clammy and horrible.

'What's the time, Sam?' said Miranda.

'Err, twenty past three.'

'I'm hungry, does anyone fancy a toastie?'

'Can we just not talk please!'

'Ooooh, so-reeee! I didn't realise you were so sensitive!'

I could hear her stage whispering in the dark to Hannibal, planning a feast.

Activity in our bed began again with renewed vigour. He did everything he'd done before but this time double speed. It was strange the way in this game it seemed that more was less somehow and that harder and faster curiously seemed to result in numb-er. After a short while he came up from the duvet and started fiddling in his trouser pockets, making a cellophane noise and later a tearing of cardboard. Sitting on the edge of the bed with his back to me, head bent in concentration, he looked careworn and I felt sorry for him for the weight of responsibility he was carrying. There was a decisive-sounding snapping noise and he turned toward me – I shut my eyes.

It is very hard for me to describe. Everything before a man is actually inside you is fun: it's playing. It can be more or less fantastic, but it's only playing. The first time a man's cock comes into you, you know it's serious, and I realised that I was out of my depth. It seemed impossible logistically. Even though he was a teenager he looked unnecessarily huge and faced with the reality of the situation I needed to say, 'I'm awfully sorry, I've made a mistake. I hadn't realised it'd be as big as this and there's no way I'm going to escape without serious injury,' but I was honour bound now. I was here and it would take me ages to get here again. I'd be in suspense, maybe for years. Besides that, I looked in his face as he positioned himself over me and he was so in earnest: eyes closed, teeth set, anxious looking, grimly dutiful even, that I didn't feel able to interrupt him.

I wanted to laugh at the madness of it! The grunting, the massive effort, but it HURT! It just wasn't going in; it didn't fit at all. I felt like I was sucking down on a drilling corkscrew. Words from the school play kept going round and round the front of my head: 'I am in blood steeped so far, that to go back is as tedious as go o'r.' I was on the verge of embarrassing us both for ever, just shouting out and pushing him off, when all of a sudden he seemed to burst in; suddenly he fitted! He relaxed onto his elbows and instead of scraping, his cock seemed to grease in and out. It was quite comforting, satisfying even.

After what seemed a very short time he appeared to electrocute himself and then flopped down, half on the bed, half on me, his face turned away but the near hand clutching a piece of fat on my hip in a companionable way.

'Thank God for that!' Suddenly Miranda's voice. 'I can get us all a sandwich. I thought it was going on for ever!'

'Not for me,' I said, my voice sounding strange. I wanted to think things over.

I must have slept, I suppose, because I don't remember anything more about their sandwich. It was just before dawn, that grey, trenches light, when he woke me again.

'Are you all right, Sue?'

I liked the way he said my name. He was leaning on one elbow, looking under the bedclothes at me. I arched my back seductively and 'ummed' a yes. He drew round my nipple with his finger dipped in spit. I moaned and tried shifting my weight from buttock to buttock a bit.

'Can we do it again?'

'Er . . . all right then,' I said.

Looking across at the other bed I could see nothing but the tops of two heads. He got up to put on a record. This time it happened to be a Mozart flute concerto. It didn't hurt the same; instead of that tearing raw burn, it was a sickly sensation, like when you dare to press a bruise. Part the way through I lost concentration, feeling Miranda's thumb gently stroking the top of my hand, finding myself echoing the speed and pressure of the movement in my own hand on Sam's spine.

But the audience participation from me was obviously too much for him as he only managed five more heaves before clinging onto me as if I was a cliff he were about to fall off, and then collapsing. I could feel Miranda's laughter through her hand as he whispered wetly in my ear, 'You didn't come that time, did you. Sorry.'

It hadn't occurred to me and I didn't have the heart to tell him just how far away I was. This time he rolled right away from me in the bed and I was able to think in peace. He hadn't fixed the replay on the record so I guess it had taken more or less the time it takes to play two movements of a Mozart flute concerto.

Miranda was busying herself with Hannibal who was invisible under the duvet. Their activity didn't seem to go anywhere this time and it was soon quiet in the room.

By now, real daylight was coming in through the curtains and the open bedroom door. White light, bluish even. It was a cold light and in it everyone seemed separate. It was no longer possible even to remember properly what had happened.

I got up, picked up my clothes and left the room. Not far away, sunlight was pouring into the conservatory where my parents would be having their first cup of tea of the day – I felt sad for them.

I didn't want to stay here anymore. There was no real breakfast anyway, only a grapefruit and some tired bananas; so I let the front door slam with great significance behind me and walked through that Sunday morning to my piano lesson.

My Road to Orgasm

MARLENE MASON

I am a thirty-eight-year-old woman who moved to Wales with my wonderful husband a decade ago. I don't know if my sexual experiences are unusual or the 'norm'. My first feelings of arousal came as a young child, although I couldn't describe what I was feeling. The first instance I remember was climbing a metal pole in a park, then sliding down. A peculiar, though not unpleasant, sensation occurred between my legs. I kept this knowledge to myself, and slid down the pole again. I think I was seven or eight.

Around this same time, one afternoon I was nosing around in a bag of old clothes and items that needed sewing, and stumbled across some hard-core pornography my father (or mother?) must have hidden. I had no idea what the people, a man and a woman attached together by a very strange looking appendage I had never seen before, were doing. I kept this to myself as well.

At the age of nine, a beautiful curly-dark-haired French girl (of course, she had to be French!) told me what 'fuck' meant. She said, 'It was when two people were married and wanted to have a baby, they did it.' I still didn't know what 'it' was exactly.

When I was twelve, a girl in my class who was rather over-developed for her age, with a 38DD chest, made fun of me because I didn't know what 'French-kissing' was. She knew. She told me she'd been 'felt up' by a fourteen-year-old boy from the local Junior High School, and she liked it. She frightened me.

I was a late bloomer, and very shy. My first French kiss was with a half-Welsh, half-Portuguese, boy with ice-blue eyes. He was two years older than me and from a different school. He was also the first boy I had sex with a few months later. I was scared, had no idea what I was doing (my parents, of course, never told me anything about sex – except I got the distinct feeling my father didn't want me to date until a reasonable age, say thirty or so). Two shocking things happened to me: I orgasmed, and, the next day, the boy came over and was crying. I'd never seen a man cry before. He was Catholic, and felt guilty for 'taking' something so precious from me. Was he using reverse psychology so I wouldn't feel bad? He also told me, later on the phone, that we shouldn't do it again as I hadn't 'come'. I was so shy, I didn't tell him the truth; I guess I 'faked' faking an orgasm! Whatever the case, we only did it two more times, and I never really felt too guilty about losing my virginity.

I think I was able to orgasm because I had masturbated some, and I knew what an 'orgasm' was supposed to feel like. Sometimes though, when I masturbated, it took forever. That was until I discovered the 'shower massage', a wonderful piece of detachable showerhead equipment with adjustable pulsating water-flow. This was much faster. I also read an excellent book by Dr Irene Kassorla called *Nice Girls Do*. This book should be required reading for all women before they lose their virginity, and required reading for all men in general.

Up until the age of twenty-two, I didn't orgasm easily during sex. I had a boyfriend who performed oral sex, and this I found was very helpful. I still would fake orgasm during sex, though, if I didn't orgasm during the actual 'penetrative' part. I'm not sure why I did this, or why any woman does this. Security, I imagine, not wanting to lose a man. Or sometimes you are tired and want to 'get it over with'. But a part of me was mad about this, how he always orgasmed and I only came about half the time. One day I decided to be honest with him. He was, needless to say, not impressed. We had a good communicative relationship, or so I thought. No man really wants to hear that his wife/girlfriend has been faking it. This didn't really help or hinder our relationship, but eventually we broke up. It wasn't until later in life that I realised he was just plain crap in bed.

Occasionally I would have an orgasm whilst sleeping. This was the most wonderful thing to me as I would wake up and want to have sex, and feel that I could orgasm very easily! Hurrah! A miraculous discovery! I read a book on lucid dreaming, and discovered that if I napped in the afternoon whilst it was light outside, and I gave myself auto-suggestion beforehand, that I would surely awaken from my nap having had a fulfilling sexual experience. It also became easier for me to orgasm in my waking life.

At the age of twenty-two, I had an epiphany. Actually, I had four orgasms in a row, something I'd never dreamed of before. My 'sexual awakening', for me even more important than losing my virginity, occurred whilst I was masturbating one evening in the bathtub: I pushed my legs up the side of the wall, and let the water run over me. I orgasmed, intensely and quite fast. I then decided to experiment, to see if I could orgasm again. I had never tried this before. (I had only orgasmed twice in the same evening with a very caring man I felt comfortable with who was excellent in bed, provided full body massage and oral sex.) I did, and again, and again. After that, it was like a floodgate opened in me, I was able to orgasm much more easily during intercourse, and actually could orgasm more than once. (I usually have to be on top, and I have to tell myself to 'let go' – silently, of course – to give in to the sensation.) From that moment on, I vowed never to fake orgasm again, and that if the man wasn't willing to put the time and effort into my pleasure as well as his, he wasn't worth my time!

Fantasies definitely help, and what fantasies!

Shit & Rainbows

CERIDWEN HUGHES

I will tell you about the rainbows first. I saw them in the air as we made love. Not entire rainbows: rainbow colours, jewel colours, sunlight-through-stained-glass-window colours. Green and blue, red and yellow and gold, shimmering in the air while I flew through pleasure, swam in joy, wet and slippery inside and out. I remember the colours pulsing, in the air and in my body; green ecstasy rippling in my vagina and in front of my eyes, blue shimmering and shining while I lay gasping and shouting with pleasure, long past thinking what his flatmates might think; long past thinking, full stop.

It was glorious. I was 33 years old and with my first lover. I had met him half a year before.

Until then, I had not had a relationship, bar a platonic loving friendship at university when I was 21, that stayed strictly above the neck and made me very happy. I didn't want sex at that time. I didn't think I ever should have sex, let alone enjoy it. I thought I'd had enough of it to last me through all the rest of my lifetimes.

Sex for me – or against me – started when I was two or three.

Impossible?

Dream on. Sexual abuse of children happens. In London and Cardiff and Llanfair-ym-Mochnant and Pwllheli and Blaenplwyf, at this moment, to a little girl or a little boy, more likely a girl.

I knew what sex was before I knew how to read or write,

only it was all the wrong sort. But there would be more than a decade of it before it stopped, and another until I began to consider that there might be good sex as well as bad, and a third before I experienced it.

I was abused by my father (a teacher) and – separately – my mother (a nursery nurse), with strict injunctions from both not to tell the other. Later they hired me out to other people for hours at a time. At eleven, I wasn't sure if I was still a child but I knew that I was a whore.

At twelve, puberty began and I knew with certainty that I was no longer a child and that being an adult was merely going to be an extension of the present, only that I was going to like what I was at present being forced to do. Everybody said so. *This is adult sex. This is what you really want and like. Look, your body is reacting.*

I hated my treacherous body that picked me up by the throat and shook me and threw me down from high mountain tops to fly through the air, fly and fly while I orgasmed against my will, until I hit the ground and shattered into a thousand pieces. I hated the body that would respond when stimulated, that would – still does – get aroused by the depiction, description or just the sheer mention of sexual violence, rape, coercion, humiliation.

I am beginning to feel turned on now, merely typing these words. It is not a feeling I enjoy, but I am beginning to learn to live with it. I'm beginning to believe that it's not my fault, and that there's nothing wrong with me. It's not the only thing that turns me on, and it's not something I ever act out or fantasise about when having sex, alone or with another.

Physical stimulation causes a physical response. If somebody sticks a pin into you, you will feel pain. If somebody forces you to ingest an emetic, you're going to throw up. You can't help it.

I've been conditioned like one of Pavlov's dogs. The trick is not to believe that nothing can be done about it, and that this is how you are.

Because something can be done about it, and this is not how I am.

I grew up in a tiny, backwards village in the early 1970s. My father thought feminism was a dirty word. My mother seemed never even to have heard it.

She was a great believer in the virgin/whore dichotomy. She did not think highly of women. Unmarried career women were, according to her, unnatural, dried-up spinsters. Sexually active ones, like a school friend of mine who had had boyfriends (not many) since she was fifteen, were 'one of those women who always need to have a man in their beds'.

I learned that whatever I would choose to do, I couldn't win.

She did not like women. I believe that she was frightened of and disgusted by female sexuality. She passed it all straight on to me. She acted out on me what had, presumably, been done to her as a little girl. It is the only explanation I can find for what she did to me, and for her marrying a pervert like my father.

She didn't like lesbians either. 'How do they know which is the male and which the female?' she asked me once after we'd watched a TV documentary on dykes together, and I daringly mentioned that I had a lesbian friend in the city where I by then lived. This was before I broke off contact with them altogether.

Lesbians puzzled her. She liked clarity: straight lines, no confusion. What stuck out of her carefully constructed black-and-white view of the world had to be removed, chopped off. She probably would have approved of cliterodectomy if it had been available in our area.

Thank the Goddess it wasn't.

Despite the sexual abuse and the large amount of damage it has done, despite both my parents' destructive attitude towards an autonomous female sexuality, somehow I am still a sexual person. I have managed to grow up to become a sexual woman.

I should like to stress that I was a sexual woman before I became a sexually active woman. It's not as though there'd been some dead wasteland between my legs before my lover came and kissed it awake.

I have always masturbated, shamefully as a teenager because the abuse – although by then over – was still so recent. I was brimful with sexual feelings that I was sure were a remnant of the abuse, as though I had been oversexed by it somehow, turned into a nymphomaniac who had to keep rubbing away the feelings that rose and rose and rose. Now I believe that I was feeling sexual because I was 14 years old and full of hormones. I was a teenager and in other, better, circumstances I should have been experimenting with my emerging sexuality, kissing and necking with boys or girls, trying out what I liked, what turned me on, what made me feel good, what gave me pleasure.

Instead I felt terrible: guilty, dirty, helpless, humiliated by the rising tide of feelings that would not stop. If I still feel like this, I thought, after all I've been through, then they were probably right, then there probably is this compulsion in me to go for what they described as 'adult sex' – abusive sex, unhealthy sex, uneven sex between non-consenting people, some adult, others not. They had told me I would graduate from being the abused to being an abuser. I wanted rather to die.

I decided not to have sex. Ever. Maybe that way I would stay safe, for myself and others.

It wasn't that I didn't sometimes, often, dream of it, but not in any realistic way. I'd dream of it, but in the knowledge that it wouldn't actually happen. I fell in love with unattainable people and backed off at the first sign that they might return my feelings.

I read lots of feminist books. I did years of therapy. I started to write again. I started to dream again.

When I was thirty I fell in love and in lust with a real person and thought that maybe, maybe, something might come of it this time. It didn't, we're not even friends anymore and she is still with her girlfriend, but for the first time I had been able to imagine myself as a real person making love with another real person. I had masturbated and thought about her and felt wonderful, and had a roaring orgasm that felt terrific. That hadn't happened before.

Maybe, maybe, I thought. One day.

Three years later, it did happen. I was seriously in love. I was seriously in lust. I left damp patches on chairs simply being in the same room with this man. He was seven years younger than me, and I thought he was gay.

I felt terrible. Not because I thought he was gay. Because I was so attracted to him when I thought I shouldn't be. I felt let down by my body which wanted, again, things I thought it shouldn't. The abuse I'd suffered as a child and a teenager had felt so terrible that I thought it should have put me off sex for life. I was afraid of my desire. All the sex I'd ever experienced had been abusive; how would I know how to make love with an equal partner? *Would* I know how to, or would I seek to replicate old patterns? How could I ever bear to have anybody look at my body? I felt fat and ugly. I was so old and so inexperienced in all but the wrong things. He would laugh. He wouldn't want me. I was an old, fat, ridiculous woman desiring a younger man.

When I masturbated, I thought of him although I tried not to. I wanted to touch him and kiss him and wind his wonderful long hair round my hands. I wanted him to make love to me, to touch my naked body.

The absolutely incredible thing was that he did, too. We were becoming friends, but there was more, somehow. And one night, we finally got round to talking about it.

Where do you want to go from here? he asked.

I didn't know how to say what I wanted. I held out my

hand and he took it. I mostly don't like people touching me, but I felt that touch all over my body, warm and sparkling like fire.

Um, I said. I don't usually fall in love with people.

Am I an exception? he asked.

Yes, I said, and felt like a slut. I'd just admitted that I wanted to go to bed with him, and I was terribly, terribly ashamed.

We kissed. I wasn't sure at first how to, and afraid I was making a fool of myself (Thirty-three and doesn't know how to kiss?) and so nervous that right away, I didn't feel anything. I said so. OK, he said, not at all put out, although his eyes were sparkling and he had a big erection and clearly enjoyed it all very much. No problem. Take a break. Don't force yourself.

We sat talking again, then sat talking holding hands, then I wanted to touch him again and feel him touch me, and a bit later we were kissing again and it felt like the most wonderful thing in the world.

We don't have to make love now, he said. I don't have any condoms, anyway.

I don't think I can, anyway, I said hastily. I . . . want to – that was so hard to say – but I've no idea how long it will take until I can. Days, weeks, months?

That's OK, he said. You set the pace. I'll follow.

We spent the rest of that night kissing, and it was like a dream. I walked home on air. It just felt so *good*. I was thirty-three, going on fifteen.

Three days later, we met up again. And kissed again. Took a few clothes off. Some hours later took a few more clothes off. Some hours later took them all off and went between the sheets because it was getting cold out. I said, I think I want to stop now; not because I wanted to but because I thought I should. Because I thought I shouldn't be enjoying this so much. I shouldn't be losing my head and getting so turned on and so, so wet.

I didn't stop.

An hour later his knee was between my legs and I was rubbing against it, while he kissed me and caressed my breasts. I thought I was flying apart with pleasure. Just the touch of his naked body on mine felt better than anything I had ever felt.

You're gorgeous, he said. Your nipples are like roses. You're very, very, very sexy.

I hadn't known anything could feel so good. I was making an indecent amount of noise. I hadn't realised how noisy I would be. Luckily, during our first few months together my partner lived in his artist's studio in a building that was completely deserted at night. By the time he moved into a flatshare we'd both got used to my acoustic explosions, and his new flatmates would have to get used to them, too.

I'd wanted the light off when we first began to make love, but as we didn't sleep at all in the beginning, dawn would creep up on us and suddenly the light was back. I didn't want him to see me, I still felt so ugly, but we'd just spent the night touching and caressing each other's bodies, and I didn't want to stop just because he could see me now. He'd felt all there was anyway. Besides, I could see him too, and that was a pleasure I didn't want to forego. So the light stayed on.

He was so beautiful. He didn't always believe me, but he was. That long white body, that long dark hair. I'd always wanted long hair and mine never grows, but now I could hide in his, fill my hands with it. After the sexual abuse, I never thought I could find an erect penis desirable, but now I did, because his felt beautiful on my hands and my tongue: so warm, so smooth. Warm silk, live silk. It jumped when I touched it. It changed all the time, turning from leathery rubber to living, breathing, warm, warm satin.

I read the Song of Solomon a lot when we first started making love. I needed something in writing to back up what I was feeling: my body singing with pleasure and my mind reeling like a bird that has just discovered flight. God knows what drove me to the Bible. But there, in the jewelled poetry of the Song of Songs, I found words for what I felt.

My beloved is white and ruddy, the chiefest among ten thousand.
His head is as the most fine gold,
his locks are curly,
and black as a raven.
His eyes are as the eyes of doves by the rivers of waters,
washed with milk, and fitly set.
His cheeks are as a bed of spices,
as sweet flowers:
his lips like lilies, dropping sweet smelling myrrh.

His hands are as gold rings set with the beryl:
his belly is as bright ivory overlaid with sapphires.
His mouth is most sweet: yea, he is altogether lovely.
This is my beloved, and this is my friend,
O daughters of Jerusalem.

I was really shocked when I found out how much I enjoyed having my vagina touched and explored and caressed and stimulated and licked and penetrated. (Isn't there a better, a positive word for this that doesn't sound like an assault?) My lover was caressing my vulva with his hand at the time, and I whispered: Just slip a finger inside me for a minute.

Just to see what that might feel like. He slipped a finger in a little way.

A bit more, I said. More. *More.* Oh, yes, *yes!*

I felt fantastic. Wonderful. Heavenly. Lustful. I was getting very noisy again.

Afterwards, I was ashamed for a week. I didn't think I should be enjoying this when the Hite Report and everyone else clearly stated that it's the clitoris where it's all at. When I masturbated by myself, it was; and my finger or a (clean, warm) candle in my vagina didn't do anything for me. But my partner's finger was an entirely different matter. I loved his finger in my cunt. I loved his tongue in my cunt. I loved his penis in my cunt.

In that order. Although one of the most wonderful sexual experiences I had was while we were fucking, the others were when his finger was in my cunt and his body alongside mine.

That's when I saw the rainbow colours in the air. I had what I believe were vaginal orgasms with him, although opinion seems divided as to whether they exist or not. I think they do. They felt like electric charges, like flying out of my body and into the stratosphere, like green and blue shimmering and shining in the air around me. I can't remember the best times, I was so far gone. All I remember is being so wet, so slippery with sweat and vaginal juices and sometimes menstrual blood, feeling better all over than I can ever put into words; shouting with pleasure, calling his name and flying, soaring, bursting with lust and with joy.

We laughed a lot. Sex can be funny.

The smacking noises a wet cunt makes.

Reddish handprints all over me, and his hand looking like the swamp thing's, because I had my period and we were both covered in menstrual blood.

We fell off the bed. It was only a single, with a wobbly mattress, and manoeuvring on it was tricky. We kept having to stop and rearrange ourselves.

My tongue went numb as I was going down on him.

I got semen in my hair.

I was kissing his belly and licking his navel, and his penis twitched and tapped me squarely on the nose.

His stubble tickled as he was going down on me, or worse, it scratched so much that I had to ask him to stop.

It could be difficult to get things right, especially to say: I'm not getting very much out of this – because it was so well meant. I didn't want to have to say, No, not, like this; not yet; try something else, faster, slower, more to the right – I wanted him to be perfect, and he wasn't. He was human, and it took me a good while to work out that that's much better than perfect, because it's real. A real, warm, live person who responded to my touch just as I did to his. Who was very relaxed and open about lovemaking, who could go off into raptures, or get the giggles with me, or be all embarrassed because he'd just assured me it was all under control and of course we wouldn't fall off the bed. Clunk.

Other things were not funny at all.

There were the memories that kept coming back just when I least wanted them. Straight flashbacks, where one minute I was in bed my with lover, here and now, feeling him and seeing him and loving him, the next I was back home, being touched up by my father or my mother or a stranger, hating it. I had to say *Stop* so often.

Once, when we were in his studio making love on a Sunday morning, a sound came from next door that sounded like a whip, and I remembered how I'd been made to hit another, naked child with a whip when I was 12, while adults were watching. I started to cry and couldn't stop.

The sound wasn't made by a whip; it was only the painter in the next studio, tacking canvas on to a frame, but it took me twenty-one years back into the past. I cried and cried and felt awful, terrible, guilty, ashamed. I was so sorry for that child, the other child whom if I'd had a choice, I wouldn't have wanted to hurt.

We had to stop making love and he held me while I cried and told me it wasn't my fault, none of it, and that I was all right and safe and grown up, and that he loved me.

After a while, I struggled back into the present and was able to feel again that I was here, not there; now, not then. I could feel that I was with a person who cared about me very much, who loved me, and whom I loved back. I was able to think that maybe, I wasn't a bad person, or not entirely. And then, that was always the joy with him, my body made itself felt. I could feel again that I was physically close to a person I loved and trusted and whose body I adored. I began to be very aware of his warm, naked skin on my warm, naked skin. We kissed, and I could almost feel my inner drawbridge going down, my pores opening, my vagina dilating and my clitoris pulsing and getting harder. I was back in the present.

Of all the miracles – they were miracles for me – that happened with this man, this was not the least: that with him, I could manage to come back from abusive past to loving present in the space of an hour or so.

The flashbacks were one of the reasons why I didn't feel able to fuck very often. It is not the sort of thing where you want to say *Stop!* half-way through. I had to feel really sure that this was what I wanted, here, now. And I didn't always trust myself. So we mostly used hands and mouths, and loved it.

There were other sorts of disturbances, as unpleasant but more insidious than the flashbacks. They would occur when I was particularly enjoying myself.

The first one happened when I was sitting on and rubbing my clitoris against my lover's thigh while he was lying back and stroking my nipples. My breasts were wobbling, I was getting up to my usual noise level and rubbing harder, when suddenly I heard my mother's voice in my ear. *Shameless*, she said. *Hussy. Whore. So this is what you're like. Shameless. Shameless.*

What I was being was unashamed. Active. Doing something purely for myself. I hadn't asked beforehand, Would you like me to do this? Would you enjoy this? I hadn't asked him to stroke my clitoris with his hand, which I knew he enjoyed.

I was doing what *I* had felt like, because it was what *I* wanted, because it felt good. Because it turned *me* on. My partner, it must be said, was getting harder by the second. But that hadn't been the point.

All of this, in my mother's book, was Hussy behaviour.

You'd think a woman who sexually abuses her own child would be above thinking in such categories, but of course she isn't. That's the whole point. If you can't live with yourself sexually, you have to find a scapegoat. If you can't acknowledge what you're feeling, you have to deny it. If the feeling gets too strong, you have to project it on to somebody else. That is how you do *not* deal with something. My mother, I think, had been abused herself as a child. It must have left her with sexual feelings she did not like and could not, as a child, cope with. When she could have coped with them as an adult, she chose not to. It wasn't as though it would have been impossible then; it was the early seventies and there were shelters, there were women's groups. She could have got away and taken me with her, even if it had meant going to Liverpool or Manchester or London, leaving her roots and her background. What is more important, your child or your status? Your life or your role as a nice respected housewife?

But she chose not to deal with it, and I became her scapegoat. I learned that sex was smutty and nasty, that when it hurt it was only what I deserved. That I was a dirty little girl for having such things done to me. That I was bringing it all on myself, and that to enjoy any of it was the worst thing of all. Enjoying sex of whatever description, even healthy, loving adult sex with a man I loved and adored and who loved and adored me, was wrong, shameless, depraved, and putting me beyond all redemption.

This was so hard to overcome, because my mother is/was (I hope she's dead) a woman. I am a woman. My body begins to look a bit like hers. It functions in the same ways that hers does. Surely being a woman, like her, I am like her in other ways?

But I'm not.

Enjoying sex is OK. I try to tell myself this, although I don't always believe it. There are still the mixed feelings: feeling turned on and nauseous at the same time, because the two went together so naturally in the past that it's sometimes difficult to remember that they're not the same thing. Feeling sexual and feeling guilty is another one, or sexual and power-less, empowered and dirty, unashamed and shameless. These are artificial combinations.

Sex is OK. Pleasure is good.

I've just said those two sentences aloud, and it is aston-ishingly difficult.

I love it when you're on top, my lover whispered when we sank from kissing upright to lie on his bed.

We have since split up, for various and complicated reasons; and I'm back to sex-for-one for the time being, which is OK and fine and can be spectacular as well, but it's not the same thing.

I miss his smile, and his eyes and his voice and his sense of humour. I miss his determination to make a way for himself in the world through his art. I miss his lovemaking and the way his skin felt on mine; his hands and his body and the little sighing noises he made in his throat when he was really turned on and loving what I was doing. I miss his touch, his mouth on my breast and his finger in my cunt.

I miss the sex.

There now. I've said it.

Loose in France

ANON

It wasn't that long ago, and I smile whenever I think about it, and blush. Not that I'm prudish, far from it. I've had some sexual escapades, believe me. But this was something else. This is not something I tell everybody, because I still can't get over the fact that it actually happened.

I was on a train, somewhere between Paris and the Alps, and I was travelling on my own. I remember exactly what I was wearing: a denim shirt with poppers down the front and a thin, light blue skirt, and matching white underwear. I always have matching underwear, just in case. And we're not talking accidents and hospitals here.

I had a carriage all to myself and I was reading by the window. It was probably something like *Paris Match* because my French was pretty rusty and badly needed a good kick up the backside before I met my friends in the South. Anyway, the sun was setting when we stopped at a station and I glanced through the window. The platform was full of French teenagers, laughing and shoving each other out of the way. My face fell. A good half dozen of them came into my carriage, so my pleasantly quiet part of the journey was over. A couple of them eyed me curiously. 'Salut,' they said.

'Salut,' I replied politely. They talked amongst themselves for a while.

They were all boys, aged from around 15 to 18 and they were members of some kind of youth club, on their way to the Alps for a week of climbing. One of their supervisors came in shortly afterwards, a very good-looking man of about 25, and asked if they were disturbing me. Not at all, I replied. That was when my rusty French accent must have betrayed me. They asked where I was from, then they asked me a few questions about rugby and the Princesse de Galles. It was all good fun and I was enjoying myself. Then one of them asked why I was on my own. I said I was going to meet some friends who lived in the Alps. So you're not married? No. Why not? Don't know, I suppose I don't feel like getting married just yet. Oh, a free spirit. Yes, you could say that. Thinking back, maybe I smiled in a certain way. I'm not sure. I certainly wasn't flirting, not consciously anyway. The boy sitting next to me was a little taller than the others, definitely older than the cheeky ones sitting opposite me, and he was quiet, shy almost. I don't think he asked me a single question, he just listened and laughed as I chatted with the younger ones.

It was late, the supervisor had gone, and a couple of the boys had nodded off. I was really tired too. There was room for me to stretch out a little on the seat, so I made a pillow out of my fleece jacket and fell asleep. I'm lucky that way – I can sleep anywhere, no problem.

Then I woke up, very slowly. I thought I was dreaming. It was dark, and I wasn't sure where I was. But there was this lovely sensation, a wonderful, gentle something happening to me. I was melting, turning to warm marshmallow. I wasn't even sure which part of me it was, to begin with. Then I realised I was in the train. I could see the vague outlines of the sleeping boys opposite me, and hear them breathing gently in the dark. And somebody was kissing my buttocks.

That's when I really woke up. But I didn't move. It felt too good. They were small, light little kisses, all over my hips, my thighs and my backside, through the thin material of my skirt. I realised with a shock that it was the tall boy who had been sitting next to me, and he was kissing me so quietly, but I could tell how excited he was. I toyed with the idea of moving, of brushing him off, so that he'd think I was still asleep, but still get the message. I didn't want to make a scene and wake up the rest of the carriage. But I didn't move, and I didn't brush him off, and I carried on pretending to be asleep. It was heavenly.

Then he became a bit more adventurous. I felt him lifting my skirt with one hand, and running the fingers of the other up my legs. Then he kissed me again, just above the elastic of my knickers. I could hardly breathe. Then he hooked his fingers in the waistband and slowly started pulling them down. I lifted my hips ever so slightly to make it easier for him, so even if he thought I was asleep before, which I doubt, he knew now that I was most definitely awake and wanting this as much as he did. And then he kissed my bare skin. Oh god, I wanted to groan, but I couldn't. The carriage was full of sleeping teenagers.

His fingers ran up my back, and round, under the front of my shirt. My nipples were like bullets, and we both moaned, ever so quietly. He played with me for what seemed like hours, and I wanted him inside me. I yearned for it. His fingers came back down, tentatively, exploring every cen- timetre of me, and he found how excited I really was. And I still hadn't moved, I'd hardly dared breathe. But he was breathing much harder now, and I could feel how hard he was. He obviously wasn't experienced, but his slightest touch was enough to bring me close. Oh. My. God. I was coming.

Then one of the young boys opposite moved, and I saw his eyes flicker open in the moonlight streaming through the window. I froze. So did my lover. He gently moved away from me, pulling my skirt back over my thighs, and I shut my eyes fiercely. I was asleep, dammit. Please think I was asleep.

We lay there for ages. My whole body was on fire. I wanted him so badly, but didn't have the guts to take him by the hand to a more private part of the train. It had been so exquisite, and the harsh lights and stale smell of a train toilet would have spoilt everything. So I smiled wantonly to myself in the dark and fell asleep.

When I woke up, the boys opposite had obviously been awake for some time and were sharing a flask of coffee. They smiled.

Bonjour. Bien dormi?

I smiled back and nodded. I sat up slowly. I didn't dare look at my neighbour. Then I realised some of my shirt buttons had come undone. I tried to close them as unobtrusively as possible, but when I looked up again, the boys had a knowing look in their eyes. Oh dear. I turned to look at my quiet young lover. He was blushing slightly, but he caught my eye and smiled.

They left at the next station, and they all waved at me through the window. I waved back. The train pulled out again, and I put my face in my hands, closed my eyes and laughed. I didn't even know his name.

20s

'But when it comes to making love –
we justify doing that in English.
After all, sex is such an 'Ych a Fi',
we couldn't possibly face each other
over the cornflakes if we did it in
our mother tongue.'

The Inconsiderate Type

ANON

Mark was good fun, sporty, intelligent and very nice to look at. Our relationship started pretty slowly with stolen glances and gentle flirting. Every time we met it progressed a stage, from snogging to a bit of coy fumbling, and finally to unreserved groping, licking and sucking. It was quite pleasant but I could tell his heart wasn't really in it. He was reluctant to touch me and pretty ineffective when he did. I wasn't surprised to hear that his previous experiences of sex were almost all drunken one night stands. As rugby captain at University, he was never short of girls keen to add him to their list of conquests. He'd take a girl to bed, climb on top of her, come, climb off and go to sleep. So he didn't quite know what to do with himself (or with me) when I wanted some sort of *foreplay*. In fact, I think he was amazed that it was possible to go to bed and not have sex.

I could cope with the lack of experience but it pissed me off that he didn't seem that interested in learning how to turn me on. He'd happily lie back and enjoy my flickering tongue, but he'd expect to follow that by pushing my legs apart and climbing aboard. Only once did he try properly to make me come. To be fair, he did give it a good go and he almost convinced me that he liked going down on me. In fact, he got me so near the brink that I shagged him in the hope of falling over the edge! I didn't reach that ultimate goal but it had definite potential. We parted fondly and with the hope of more of the same.

Unfortunately, I then had to go away for a month. When I returned, I was feeling really horny and looking forward to a good shag. I was keen to get naked and sexy, but when I saw Mark he just didn't do it for me. I'd hoped my affectionate feelings for him would re-emerge and we'd do the boyfriend-girlfriend thing, but he bored me and the sex was absolutely awful. When I first arrived at his house, we stripped off and things proceeded very quickly. Neither of us bothered much with foreplay this time, and soon his naked bottom was flashing around the room as he searched frantically for a condom. I'd have thought he'd have had the foresight to put one near to the bed, but no, he had to wade through cupboards, drawers and finally his wash bag before he emerged with a precious little square packet!

Things didn't get any better when we couldn't put it on properly and our rubber friend ended up in a heap on the floor. This somewhat interfered with our excitement. Condom number two (from a drawer this time) was force-fed on by Mark and we spent the next five minutes trying to get the damn thing inside me. Once inside, and almost hard, we stuck to the one position for not very long. Then with almost no build up he was getting off me and that was, very disappointingly, that.

The next morning, Mark made a brief attempt to excite me with his hand. When I was bored, I suggested another condom. At least I could take control and perhaps get some excitement that way. His reaction was, 'It would all be over very quickly if we got a condom,' and he took his hand away from me completely. I was very frustrated by this but continued to wank him off while I decided what to do next. My mind was already concluding that this relationship wasn't going to work when he perked up with, 'I know it's really selfish to ask, but can I have a blowjob?'

'Fuck off, you haven't done anything for me,' was not my most considered response, but I was horrified. Amazingly, he wasn't deterred by my venom and he asked me again a few minutes later. 'Oh go on. Please can I have a blow job.'

I knew then that the relationship was over, but I obliged his request so that I could end the sexual part as soon as possible, without completely severing our friendship. When he came, I jumped off the bed like a rocket and spat out his horrible sperm noisily into the sink. In some ways, it felt quite good to reject him so violently, but the childish satisfaction didn't come close to making up for his awful attitude. That was it.

Before my month away, I had been quite happy to 'teach' Mark how to turn me on, and to educate him that women like a little more than a quick imprecise grope and to give blow-jobs. I'd hoped that he could learn to give me orgasm after mind-blowing orgasm. But suddenly, now, it hit me across the face that it really wasn't worth the bother. Mark might try to excite me every now and again but he'd never enjoy it. Sex for him had never been much more than wanking made easy, and that wasn't going to change. If he touched or licked me first then it would be a means to an end and not part of the pleasure. I need to feel wanted, desired and an essential part of the whole process. No, the relationship would never work. Some men like exploring women's bodies and some don't. Mark doesn't. It's as simple as that.

Sex Would Probably be Fantastic . . .

ANON

Sex would probably be fantastic if I wasn't constantly worried that my hair will resemble Worzel Gummidge and my make-up Aunt Sally before, during and after the event. I don't know how it feels to be confident and to have that wonderful couldn't-care-less attitude about your body. Don't get me wrong. I am not one of those women who can't even go to the toilet without putting her face on; in fact if you gave me a lip liner I'd probably try and poke my eye out with it, but I do think it must be wonderful really to not worry about anybody else's opinion.

If you look back on your childhood there are probably clues: like the fact that girls play with Barbie dolls. With the best will in the world very few of us will ever share her vital statistics. If occasionally she came with stretch marks, droopy boobs and a bum that skimmed the top of her perfect thighs maybe we could all start feeling better about ourselves. It hardly seems fair when boys have Action Man as a role model. Have you ever noticed how Action Man always has to have something in his hand? Good move because I am sure that most of us are aware that if a man has nothing in his hand he can't seem to stop checking that his bits and bobs are still there. I wonder how it would look if women were constantly clutching themselves. Probably as though the entire female population were desperate for the loo! Getting back to Action Man, you only have to look at the size of his tools to realise why most men think that anything longer than a fingernail means they are some kind of Sex God. Not much scope for disappointment there.

Personal appearance aside there is something about sex with a stranger that has a more raw, animal feel about it than when you are suffocating under feelings of love and commitment. I think one of my most memorable experiences was with a complete stranger in the front of a car. Perhaps the fact that I was anonymous helps; I know that Rachel the nurse was a lot more exciting than the real me. Needless to say the man in question had consumed a large amount of alcohol and was probably completely oblivious to this wild woman I had unleashed for the occasion, but it did wonders for my confidence. I seem to recall that he even paid me a compliment about my enormous nipples. I didn't have the heart to tell him that actually that wasn't just my nipples, more my entire breast. When you are a 32aa you don't get many compliments aimed at your chest area. In fact, when you are a 32aa you don't get many compliments full stop. Funny that!

In short, I feet that sex is something we all feel we should enjoy but only a select few seem to manage it on a regular basis. I'm sure a lot of women would far sooner have a bar of chocolate any day. If you speak openly to women in a steady relationship a large proportion will openly admit to faking orgasms simply to speed up the process. Very few men can resist the animal screams of a pleasured woman.

Maybe if men were a little more romantic and imaginative we wouldn't have to be such good actresses. I'm sure that they believe they are being erotic, but do they realise how painful it is to have your nipples twisted round or to have an entire hand shoved between your legs? There was one guy who, I swear, wasn't going to be happy until he had both hands inside and was able to clap along to his favourite tune. Not my idea of fun.

To end I think it is only fair to say that men are probably just as insecure as we are about sex but perhaps their animal instinct and desire to do what comes naturally is greater than their insecurities. One thing is for certain: if a man rolls over and asks how it was for you, either get a new boyfriend or perfect your acting skills. Better still, leave them guessing; they may try harder next time.

A Decade of Fumbling

ADELE WOODS

He lay there, trembling like a leaf. I couldn't believe it. After all the times he'd asked for this, asked me to have sex with him, and now that I'd decided the time was right, he was shaking. We fumbled onwards anyway. We were both virgins, neither of us really knew what we were doing. My sex education from school had been forgettable. *More* magazine and *Just Seventeen* were infinitely more useful. I didn't ask about his. Probably just as well, since I later found a porn magazine under his bed, the photographs depicting women in chains. I know now that my early attempts at sex were driven by curiosity rather than lust. The relationship didn't last long. It was always on and off. He lacked the maturity necessary for a relationship, despite ironically, possessing the necessary sexual maturity.

My second boyfriend was far more confident about his sexuality. Unfortunately this didn't rub off on me. As a result of his attitude to sex, I was left feeling unsure and ashamed of my sexual behaviour. He didn't believe in sex before marriage. That was fine, he didn't have to sleep with me. However, that wasn't the problem. He found it unforgivable that I'd already lost my virginity, and somehow, somewhere on the college grapevine, he heard that I'd 'done it' with my first boyfriend nine times. Not a mistake then! He condemned my earlier behaviour, even going so far as to suggest I was a slut in letters he sent me. Ironically enough our rumblings under the sheets in the spare room at his house, when things were still good between us, were full of sexual tension. It was never safe to completely undress and we'd remove the odd garment here and there or unbutton a shirt for easier access. Perhaps it was the thrill that we might be discovered, or just first lust, but he gave me my first orgasm, and only orgasm so far.

I got lucky with the third boyfriend. We were even engaged until he left me. He understood that people fall in and out of love, and in and out of bed, with other people. He was my first experience of good sex, sex that was free of guilt or shame. For the first time I was free to experiment with somebody else who was just as keen as me. We tried different positions, we made love on the sofa, I shared my first bath with a man, and I even dressed up for him. I was fortunate enough to be able to fit into my school P.E. kit, that I'd last worn at the age of thirteen. I desired him but I loved him as well. He instilled sexual confidence in me, at least whilst I was with him, and until I slowly lost it again.

When I got to university in Wales, I discovered a wild streak in me. First time away from home, and some heavy drinking, led to my first one-night stand. Well, actually, it was two one-night stands, but with the same bloke. Can I still call that a one-night stand? I was snogging him in the Quarry, carried away by the incredibly bad live band. It was definitely lust, we made love three times each night, but it was also a painful lesson in men's double standards. He was just using me and I was too naive to know that I should be using him too. Despite encouraging me to go all the way, he was quick to tell me later that you shouldn't sleep with a man on a first date. He also had an incredibly high opinion of himself. When he was sat naked on my bed, he told me that I'd probably be selling my story to the papers in a few years time. I'm still waiting . . .

That episode deterred me for a couple of months. I concentrated on studying and getting drunk instead. Eventually, the next one came along. He was in my seminar group. We were discussing the Irish question, some participating quite wholeheartedly in the debate. Then he piped up, with his charming Irish accent, and suddenly people were less keen to air their views. It must have been his voice, that beautiful accent, that turned my head. It was enough to make me desire him. Yet when I had him there, to myself, I found that I didn't want him at all. The sex was cold, mechanical and performed almost dutifully. Needless to say the liasion only lasted a couple of weeks.

I found even less sexual inspiration in my next union, the longest relationship of my life to date. He was a virgin and, therefore, wanted me to take control. I felt hopeless, and the sexual side of things never went right from the start. I wanted him to inspire me, to take over. I'm so easily distracted. I knew I needed a strong lover, not someone so shy and unsure. We rarely made love in the first couple of years and later on not at all. By the end of it I couldn't bear him to touch me. I could arouse him, but I couldn't arouse me. My mind wasn't remotely turned on, or tuned in. Whilst I was with him I even began to doubt my sexual desire. Was I frigid or devoid of sexual feeling? It was lucky for me that we split up briefly in middle of our time together when I met an older man. Perhaps he was fated to come into my life, to remind me of my sexual desire, to reawaken it in me.

It's funny, but looking back I think I understand him better now than I did when I was twenty. He was thirteen years my senior. Mum disapproved. During our first fateful date in The King's Head, the sexual attraction was irresistible. We had to leave the pub and retreat to the privacy of my hall room because we couldn't stop kissing. I had never felt such a strong desire for someone. He would have had me there and then if he'd have had a condom on him. He lived in a village near Tregaron, and all our further meetings took place there. I loved the isolated feel of the place, and the house was so big and old fashioned. He took a real delight in my body and even in the short time that I was with him, taught me a lot about making love. There was still a part of me that was afraid to let go, so I took a perverse delight in being told I was a naughty girl, and shyly enjoyed being soaped down in his bath tub. I left him because I still loved my previous boyfriend, and because I could see no future in the relationship. I was close to finishing my final exams and, therefore, close to leaving Wales.

Returning to Wales, aged 22, I met the man with whom I was to share my longest sexual relationship. Again, in the security of a longer relationship I was free to develop a real intimacy and use this as a springboard for sexual exploration. Luckily the skirt of the P.E. kit had one of those adjustable waists. To begin with, I think he was slightly nervous about his sexual prowess. He always came very quickly and by his own admission had a small willy. These things weren't important to me. I always wanted him, was always thinking about being in bed with him, or on the floor with him, or even over the kitchen table. My mind used to wander terribly in exams with thoughts of him. Over time I became aware that the sexual side of the relationship, indeed the whole relationship was more important to me than him.

When I lost him I spent a few months regaining my independence, and finding 'me' again. My period of solace was followed by an ill-judged love affair with someone who had admired me years before. Only three and a half years had passed but I found him different in the most important ways. I no longer really desired him. I'd always been afraid that I'd just been flirting with him from the safety of a relationship, knowing it would never go any further. Now it was for real, I found he didn't particularly interest me. The sex was again performed dutifully with no real pleasure. I found his work ethic overbearing and we parted ways.

They say you should never have a sexual relationship with one of your work colleagues. Well, you know, it wasn't meant to happen. I'd never thought about him that way, until he took my number, met me for a drink, and got talking. I found him charming, funny, and just such good company. By arousing my mind, he aroused my body. The second time we went out I got us both drunk, almost deliberately, and had to take him back to my flat, as it was nearer than his place. We made love. With him it was always 'making love', rather than shagging or fucking, or just fumbling in the dark. His body was beautiful. He was a good size. He gave me something to grab hold of, without being overweight. His skin was a gorgeous bronze colour and he had wiry black hair all over his chest that spiralled downwards towards his cock. His eyes twinkled and his teeth were so white, making his smile a little alarming in the middle of the night. He was a good lover, my best lover, he made all the right moves in all the right places. He had the social skills and grace as well. In the beginning he never failed to tell me I was gorgeous or pass some admiring comment on my clothing.

However, he's not the relationship type. That knowledge in itself has led me to assess the way I lead my sexual life. He inspired me to look beyond the conventions of society. Why do people try to be faithful to one another when it's just not a part of human nature, and why do people marry so young? Why marry at all? We can admit that we too have sexual desires and discover them and develop our desires without being ostracized or punished by society. Convention no longer requires women to marry. We don't live in an age of chastity. Food for thought. So, following this, I undertook my last sexual adventure with a pinch of salt, which was just as well really. Four dates and three shags, and I don't think he'd ever heard of foreplay. I'll stick to my non-committal Spanish lover and keep my independence thank you very much. I think that's called having your cake and eating it.

Sex in a Strange City

SIAN MELANGELL DAFYDD

Something, deep down was wrong. The deepest you can get in a woman is her womb, because men don't go there. And there, I felt something was missing.

Think for a second. There's a reason why I'm typing away at my laptop about the most passionate subject in my heart and bones, in a language that isn't my own. Again, I ask, what's a 'womb' in Welsh? Here lies the problem. Apparently it's 'croth' but I thought that was something biblical that only Mary had. 'Vagina', now that's another matter. We Welsh, you know – we call our vagina by all sorts of things. When my friend Sara was eleven, she got terrified when hairs started growing on her 'Jemima' – and I thought 'Puddleduck'. Your 'Jemima' should have feathers, not hairs. Then she showed me. We had just been swimming in the lake, and tried to get changed in the passenger seat of our fathers' cars. She wanted to know that everyone else's was growing too and wouldn't believe that mine wasn't. Considering that I'm older and all. So she said we should both show, together. There she was, sat on the leather, with her flowered knickers to one side, and me stood behind the open door of the car, hiding from everyone else. So we stuck our naked vaginas out, facing each other and wondered at our differences. Her knickers were prettier. Behind my knickers, I had smooth skin, and she had a balding head look, with just the few dark hairs. We both got embarrassed at our difference and covered up, in case someone found out what we were sharing. I started to understand.

When she was sixteen, her Clint (Eastwood) gave her an 'Orange' for the first time, when she was in the bath. Figure that one out if you can.

We might complain if someone has 'chips' for dinner instead of its rightful Welsh name, or 'baked beans' with a plateful of other Welsh named food, but when it comes to making love – we justify doing that in English. After all, sex is such an '*Ych a Fi*' disgraceful thing, we couldn't possibly face each other over cornflakes if we did it in our mother tongue. 'Vagina' is something that goes by the name of 'Red Sleeve' because, you see, we women are terrifying creatures that truly belong on the film set of *Aliens*. Hang around too close and an extra arm will reach out of our deep, mysterious 'hole' and aim for your throat, punch you, leave slime all over you. Or maybe this name is the linguistics pennyworth for the cause, to make all women more like men, and give them too a dangly thing between their legs. Don't you think that she would be easier to understand if she had at least a pretend penis, even if it's a knitted sleeve thing?

I hate to dispel the myth, but, just for the record, vaginas are not knitted. So let me tell you about one man who made me look for a corner in this world where women, or specifically this woman here – I – am worth touching. This man was only sixteen, so call him a man only if you feel that it's a fitting description. He was named after a king, and liked it. He had stubble, and liked that too, though he complained about the constant shaving, and scratched his chin, to point out that he was a man. He never touched any part of me other than my lips and made sure he took out his chewing gum before doing that. After a week of this body-avoiding, he turned around to me, at the back seats of a Town Hall, the night of the Young Farmers Eisteddfod, and said, 'I want to sleep with you,' twice, aloud.

I pretended not to hear, but a few people around us heard, twice, and made big eyes at him, whilst he just sank into his seat and squeezed his cock tight to pretend it was never there.

Then he pretended not to see me for a while until I got the message and I saw him touching lips like a well-engineered bridge, bums apart, with a another girl, woman, whatever, who obviously wasn't worth touching completely either.

That was the beginning of the relationship my bum had with mid air, since sex you see, isn't about touching. It's about isolating pieces of yourself like pebbles off a rock, and giving those away to be juggled by someone whilst keeping the rest of yourself cool, calm and collected. When I ate a mango in the bath, it was more like what I wanted sex to be, licking the juice from my elbow to my little finger, ripping lightly at the flesh and licking the core stone. My tongue knew it so well, I thought I could mould it if I was blind. Maybe my mango was one step from being one of Sara's 'Oranges'. I let the mango slip, cold along the hot water on my skin, but I wasn't quite fulfilled.

I went away. You could call it running away, but I'll say this much – it was to a hot city. I didn't know this until I landed. I found myself in a place that had an entire new language, one that covered greetings, bread-buying, rail-ticket-buying and sex. As the aeroplane was about to land, I wondered, how on earth do the people of this country earn a reputation for being such passionate beings? The fields were exact squares. It was a maths paper with shy grass, and I had nothing but a sudden understanding of Welsh Mountains, like voluptuous naked sleeping women. The 'passionate' place seemed just limp. We landed into heat. That was the key. Looking at the amazing jigsaw of people, buses, junk stalls, exhaust fumes, me, and sticky ice cream holding the whole picture together, I wondered how it all fitted into one public square. Sitting on a bus, waiting for water, my skin started to change, open to the heat. Do you have a favourite word, for the sound of it, I mean? Say it slow – isn't 'heat' entrancing? It feels as if you are breathing out heat as you say it, and that's how I felt. Not until then did I remember where these peoples' passion came from. It's from heat. And so I sat on my luggage in a ball, resting my lips on my arm and looking over it like over a hill. The feeling of being on the road like that is the same as feeling undressed, bare to the minimum – nothing left but the jewellery that won't come off my fingers, even in cold water, just me. So, in the heat, I felt my own tongue in my mouth. The alien air around me made me feel everything much closer, as if every nerve ending bud had just opened, and I was being kissed, always, over and over, constantly.

It was in this city that I met a man, who I've decided, should remain nameless. So let's call him 'September', since that's when it was. It's a strange time of year, when the buildings stubbornly hold onto the summer heat from the odd cold-ish day attempting to drag it out of them. For the most part, the buildings win the day, and heat seems to radiate out of the city's edges. People still wear a look of exhaustion, as if they've collapsed into the street after having just finished making love to summer, still wearing next to nothing and glowing with an ice-cream-smelling sweat. It was with strawberry and pistachio stickiness on my lips I met September in a tall and narrow street after watching a film I wouldn't otherwise have watched.

The film was *Priscilla, Queen of the Desert* and I loved, loved and stayed fascinated by it, knowing that there were people in the audience getting plenty of Sara's 'Oranges' from it. It had all been a mistake. There was a man whose name I never knew imitating a mosquito and insisting on pinching my bum in the street, so I sneaked into this nice airy cinema to escape. I had sunk into my seat successfully, the little Methodist beast in me dragging even my split ends into the lumpy cushion of the seat whilst whispering, 'You're not really here, and nobody will see you here, in a place like this,' drag, drag. But it was all too late, because I still watched. It was the same little beast who tippex-ed all the sexy words out of the Welsh dictionary, but was failing miserably at making me invisible, because I had to walk out of the cinema, on two feet somehow, and I'm a visible 5"7'. It was at that exact moment September's voice made me turn around.

He was a clean and dirty man, all in one. He looked clean and scrubbed, but with the odd scratchy lump of clay hardened onto him, clinging. I thought straight away of my attempt at love with the man named after a king, and our failure to *cling*. This man had got it. It was lunchtime, and just outside the cinema hall, there was a food stall. We ate in the street. He was a sculptor. He moulded a piece of bread between the thumb and finger of his right hand, at the same time moulding another piece with his tongue. I think back, and I think, 'I do not, under any circumstance, trust strange men, I do not take sweets from strangers. What were you thinking, girl, you idiot!'

But I didn't take anything from him, and I was travelling so there somehow wasn't any concept of not moving on. We rambled, we ate, and in a small public square round the corner, he had a studio with big glass doors onto the street that seemed to let the breeze in and not the heat, which was by then at its height, at midday.

Men on bikes slowed down to see inside. I can tell you that because I spent enough time in there. On the far wall there was a 'chaise longue' smelling of toasted sunflower seeds, and which made puffs of dry clay clouds every time I rearranged myself on it. It started clinging to me. September was working on something marble and I just read and wrote letters, and noticed the world going by from left to right and right to left through to the doors in front of me. That didn't last long.

Mid-carving a delicate finger, September threw a blanket on top of the marble and said that something was wrong, that something was missing. Well I knew that! I knew that there was more to kissing than touching lips, that my whole body should be in it, not left untouched and empty. September started touching it. He got hold of a dollop of clay and got stuck into it until I could almost feel my fingers turning into clay to finger his – but I was turning the pages of a book, peering up at him and watching.

'You have inspired me!' he said. I translate, of course. 'I must make something else.' His finger gave a lump of clay a sort of belly button and I stayed there, lounging, wondering how he could sculpt my belly button, being that it was hidden under a vest top. But it was mine. You could only just make me out, but it was me, my belly, the turn of it, and he was stroking it into place, going in and out, reaching right in there into where my womb would be and stroking even that. I grew in front of my eyes, and he held me, he held all around me to sculpt the back of my shoulders as if that was the only way he could make them, by feeling them, as if he was used to holding me like that. His finger trailed up the centre of my back, tickling that little dip all the way up. At a glance, he had known my body well enough to sculpt me, without sight. It was scary, and seductive. When he leaned away from moulding my back, my body's clay left dark red stains on his T-shirt and arms. He was holding me so close, and did everything by pressing against me.

I made myself more comfortable and lay watching, book dropped, spine upwards. I swear he didn't have to keep sculpting me, that I was looking all right the first time, but he kept on caressing me, making sure. It might not have been necessary, but it was fun anyway. He smiled from behind my bum and smoothed it over with eight fingertips, playing a cheeky peep-o.

I wanted him to get to my breasts. I wanted him to stroke my collar bone from right to left as light as a necklace, as light as the jewellery that won't come off my body even in cold water. And finally, he did it, he cupped clay in one slow movement, and I appeared from under his palm, one and two breasts, erect after wanting to appear for so long. That was not enough. I knew that this body he was attending to, the whole body was mine, but he still worked at it. With every movement, I could almost, and I say almost because I tingled, I almost felt his sliding fingertips around, and then pulling my nipples up and hard, into shape.

The torso he created had no head. He hadn't created lips. The sculpture could not kiss. Four hours passed too quickly. I felt like he was playing a game, and had no idea where it was leading. Checking my belly button again, inspecting it, he bumped his cheek against my breast and a piece of me was left there, clinging to him. Was he gay? Was he just not turned on by what he had in his fingers, beyond me being more interesting than an apple and orange? I pressed my vagina against the clay of the 'chaise longue' just to keep myself still. Then, after inspecting my clay belly button, he looked up at my eyes behind his image of me, and, with no warning, without looking at the sculpture, created in two quick swoops, my vagina and inner thighs, so I nearly bit my lower lip off with, oh I don't know – such maddening pleasure, and failure to keep it for more than a milli-second. Go back there!

But he was done. The sculpture was a finished piece. He left only one fingerprint on me – and that was on a curl of hair that he moved out of my face's way to say good bye, and thank me for the inspiration. He hugged me closer than anybody had ever kissed me, and I had found what I was looking for. I had found being with someone in my entirety, touching every surface of my body with his – but I was still waiting to feel it! Jealous of a sculpture of myself, I left and clay stuck a clump of my hair into a curl.

Back in an empty Youth Hostel above a cafe, early evening and a roomful of white beds, with breeze and open shutters, my legs separated, my arms separated, my hips yearned upwards, and I had one thin white sheet over me. I felt myself as if my fingers were September's, and moulded away. OK, so sometimes I thought that I might be interrupted.

But really, I stopped being shocked and forgot being silly and found that right where September had last stroked the sculpture of me, my vagina needed more moulding. There, pressing my body right against September's heat, I mixed the sweat that we created like clay and clung to him. Again, I could feel him holding me like he held my image, all around, bums in, crutches tight. No oranges here, no mangoes, only orgasms, and sweeter! There, with the sour smell of coffee from downstairs dying, I wondered at how sweet the sex of one woman could smell all by herself.

Notes on Contributors

Anne-Ruth Alton was born in 1952 in Manchester and lived for many years in the north-west of England. She now lives in south-west Wales. She has been writing 'more off than on' for over forty years and comments: 'It's been said that the most difficult journey is the one from the armchair to the computer. Once I make it I'm fine, but oh, the getting there!'

Her short stories have appeared in small press magazines and she teaches Creative Writing for the Open College of the Arts. She has an MA in English Literature and Philosophy.

Elizabeth Baines was born in Bridgend and now lives in Manchester. She is the author of numerous published short stories and the novels 'The Birth Machine' (Starling Editions) and 'Body Cuts' (Pandora). She is also an award-winning radio playwright. Her prize-winning stage play 'O'Leary's Daughters' was performed at the Barons Court Theatre, London, in November 2003. Her website is at www.elizabethbaines.com.

Anne Colledge was born in Ruabon but now lives not far from the Angel of the North in beautiful, wild, north-east England, which is so often called 'The Secret Kingdom'. She has five grandchildren, two in UK and three in the USA. This keeps her busy travelling to visit them all. She likes to kayak, cycle and reads a lot. Her house is full of books. She loved teaching deaf children, which she did for thirty years. Now she has more time to write and her last book for children, 'Northern Lights', published by Piper's Ash Ltd, has a deaf hero. Her website is at www.annecol.co.uk.

Sian Melangell Dafydd lives in Cardiff with a left-hand drive Fiat Seiccento whose Italian numberplate was BR 26ORE (26 hours) – making Sian the lucky one with an imaginary extra two hours a day to write. Originally from Bala, Gwynedd, she read History of Art at the University of St Andrews and is now the Marketing Manager for Wales' new writing company, Sgript Cymru. She finds herself living in her capital city via a career taking her to Flowers East Gallery, London and Sol Sculpture Park, Tuscany where she happened on those precious extra 2 *ore*!

Gwerfyl Delahaye is a pseudonym.

Katherine Downham is a pseudonym.

Melanie Glyn is a pseudonym.

Vron Gregg is a pseudonym.

Ceridwen Hughes is a pseudonym.

Sue James is a pseudonym.

Sarah Jones is a pseudonym.

Ruth Joseph grew up in Cardiff and dreamt of writing fiction while working for IPC magazines as a freelance journalist. She is now completing her M. Phil. In Creative Writing at Glamorgan University. A Rhys Davies competition prize winner and Cadenza prize winner, she has had work accepted by Honno Modern Fiction, Accent Press, Loki Books, New Welsh Review and Cambrensis. She is now working with a film company to adapt one of her short stories for film. She is encouraged and inspired by husband, son, daughter, son-in-law and most beautiful granddaughter.

Marlene Mason was born and raised in the Pacific Northwest of America and has lived in Wales for the last decade with her husband. She works as a funding officer, bringing much-needed extra money into Wales for projects for special educational needs and young people facing barriers. Her writing has appeared in various magazines and she is currently at work on a literary-comedic novel based on her travels in Europe and the Middle East.

Suzee Moon is a pseudonym.

Jill Teague was born and brought up in the Rhondda. She studied English Literature at Swansea University. Having taught English for many years in Hampshire and Yorkshire she has now relocated to Wales. She spends half the year in the Rhondda and half in a cottage in Snowdonia. 'Twelve Trees' is her first completed piece of prose writing. She is currently working on a poetry anthology, 'Turning the Leaf', and a collection of stories entitled 'The Indigo Bowl'.

Alice Winter is a pseudonym.

Adele Woods is a pseudonym.

ABOUT HONNO

Honno Welsh Women's Press was set up in 1986 by a group of women who felt strongly that women in Wales needed wider opportunities to see their writing in print and to become involved in the publishing process. Our aim is to publish books by, and for, women of Wales, and our brief encompasses fiction, poetry, children's books, autobiographical writing and reprints of classic titles in English and Welsh.

Honno is registered as a community co-operative and so far we have raised capital by selling shares at £5 a time to over 350 interested women all over the world. Any profit we make goes towards the cost of future publications. We hope that many more women will be able to help us in this way. Shareholders' liability is limited to the amount invested, and each shareholder, regardless of the number of shares held, will have her say in the company and a vote at the AGM. To buy shares or to receive further information about forthcoming publications, please write to Honno:

'Ailsa Craig'
Heol y Cawl
Dinas Powys
Bro Morgannwg
CF64 4AH.